Stronger After Stroke

Stronger After Stroke
Your Roadmap to Recovery

Third Edition

Peter G. Levine

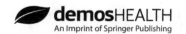

demosHEALTH
An Imprint of Springer Publishing

Visit our website at www.springerpub.com

ISBN: 9780826124135
e-book ISBN: 9780826124715

Acquisitions Editor: Beth Barry
Compositor: diacriTech

Medical information provided by Demos Health, in the absence of a visit with a health care professional, must be considered as an educational service only. This book is not designed to replace a physician's independent judgment about the appropriateness or risks of a procedure or therapy for a given patient. Our purpose is to provide you with information that will help you make your own health care decisions.

The information and opinions provided here are believed to be accurate and sound, based on the best judgment available to the authors, editors, and publisher, but readers who fail to consult appropriate health authorities assume the risk of injuries. The publisher is not responsible for errors or omissions. The editors and publisher welcome any reader to report to the publisher any discrepancies or inaccuracies noticed.

Library of Congress Cataloging-in-Publication Data

Names: Levine, Peter G., author.
Title: Stronger after stroke : your roadmap to recovery / Peter G. Levine.
Description: Third edition. | New York : Demos Health, an imprint of Springer
    Publishing Company, LLC, [2018] | Includes bibliographical references and
    index.
Identifiers: LCCN 2018000373| ISBN 9780826124135 | ISBN 9780826124715 (ebook)
Subjects: LCSH: Cerebrovascular disease. | Cerebrovascular
    disease—Patients—Rehabilitation. | Self-care, Health.
Classification: LCC RC388.5 .L48 2018 | DDC 616.8/1—dc23
LC record available at https://lccn.loc.gov/2018000373

Contact us to receive discount rates on bulk purchases.
We can also customize our books to meet your needs.
For more information please contact: sales@springerpub.com

Printed in the United States of America by McNaughton and Gunn.
18 19 20 21 22 / 5 4 3 2 1

Contents

Foreword

You are likely reading this book because someone you love has had a stroke, or you are researching the topic of stroke on your own behalf. Either way, you have made an important first decision: to focus on *recovery* rather than *compensation*. How are these concepts different?

If you choose *compensation*, you choose to use the stronger side of your body and capitalize on what you are currently able to do. A focus on *recovery* means that the activities you do are directed toward restoration of your former abilities. Focusing on recovery is hard work and underpins the treatments outlined in this book. Directing your energies toward recovery means that you always try to use your weaker side first. Humans are optimizers; we are successful in the world because we use the abilities we have to their full potential. It is normal to use your stronger side after a stroke; however, consider that neuroplasticity is abundant especially in the first six months after a stroke. If you repeatedly use your stronger side to complete your activities of daily living, neuroplasticity will be used to make your stronger side stronger and more coordinated, while making your weaker side weaker (a process known as learned nonuse—explained fully in this book).

As a neurological physical therapist, neuroscientist, and stroke researcher, I appreciate the quality of the message and the scope of the research distilled in this third edition of *Stronger After Stroke* by Peter G. Levine. Pete has provided a field manual that outlines concrete steps you can take to foster better recovery. You are unique, your brain is unique, and your stroke is unique. Read the book, consider the advice of others, and try things out. Recognize that progress may be slow and some techniques will work better for you than other techniques.

This book is a good resource for extra therapy ideas so you can capitalize on neuroplasticity. As you read and re-read sections of this book, consider the high levels of practice required to gain plasticity-driven proficiency in the movements you are practicing. Remember "practice makes permanent," so when well-meaning family and friends offer to help, show them this book and encourage them to join you as rehabilitation partners and movement coaches.

Michelle Ploughman, BSc.PT, MSc, PhD
Canada Research Chair (Tier II); Rehabilitation,
Neuroplasticity and Brain Recovery
Assistant Professor, Physical Medicine & Rehabilitation
Faculty of Medicine, Memorial University of Newfoundland

Preface

I wrote this book because I couldn't figure out why it hadn't already been written. *So much* has been discovered about recovery in the last two decades, but the information wasn't getting to survivors. If you search magazines and the Internet you might get a smattering of related information, but there was no singular source. *Stronger After Stroke* is a "field manual" of information unifying and simplifying *most* of what is currently known about recovery. The word *most* is emphasized because one of the clear messages of this book is held within the proverb: "Give a man a fish, feed him for a day. *Teach* a man to fish and feed him for a lifetime." Recovery requires knowing the latest and greatest research. The Resources section includes quick and easy ways of discovering what is new and effective in stroke recovery research.

Billions have been spent on stroke recovery research. You should benefit.

The first edition of *Stronger After Stroke* (2008) had a simple message: *When it comes to recovery, stroke survivors are in control.* Only survivors can leverage the power of brain plasticity for recovery. *Stronger After Stroke* wasn't the first source to advocate a "neuroplastic model of stroke recovery." It was, however, the first to pull the idea from scientific journals and books, explain it so everyone could understand it, and bundle it with tools survivors could use. The second edition expanded the same theme. This third, fully revised and updated new edition continues this tradition with new insights from psychology, psychiatry, rehabilitation science, exercise science, and, most importantly, neuroscience. But don't blink. Scientists from around the world are adding their voices and expanding our understanding of how to rewire to recover. To catch a glimpse of this ever-expanding perspective, have a look at this book's companion website (**Google: Stronger After Stroke blog.**)

Beyond the science, there is a very human aspect to the information in this book. I have done hundreds of talks across the United States, many at the most respected rehabilitation hospitals in the United States. Ideas are exchanged with thousands of therapists during these talks. Many of the ideas in this book reflect those discussions—their best ideas for recovery, presented to you.

It is clear that stroke survivors have taken the message this book presents to heart. And the message is spreading— since the first edition it has been translated into several languages. *Stronger After Stroke* has also changed the way stroke is talked about, and it's easy to track its influence. Prior to the publishing of the first edition, people who had a stroke were written about in the press (popular and scientific) as either *patients* or *victims*. When I wrote the first edition I knew many survivors who were neither patients nor victims, and reflected that by exclusively using the word *survivors*. Now survivors are almost always referred to as *survivors*. There have been other concepts from *Stronger* that have been generally accepted by both survivors and clinicians. Some examples are deemphasizing the plateau, focus on brain plasticity, the neuroplastic model of spasticity reduction, etc.

There has been another phenomenon surrounding this book as well: plagiarism. Either word for word plagiarism, or as a sort of reverse engineering of the whole sections of the book. Even the title has been ripped off. Since the first edition the Journal of the American Academy of Neurology, University of Tennessee Medical Center, and Emerson Hospital, and many others have all called articles in print or on line "Stronger After Stroke."

The fact that this book has a big footprint is a good thing because I have only one hope for this book.

I hope it helps.

HOW FASCINATION WITH THE BRAIN HAS HELPED SURVIVORS

Hippocrates was the first to define stroke—2,400 years ago. For most of the time since, rehabilitation was a patchwork of techniques based on clinical expertise and educated guesses. Within the last couple of decades, these techniques have been forced to give way to rigorous scientific consideration. Sheer curiosity has driven scientists to stroke recovery. Recovery from stroke provides a unique perspective on the capability of the brain. And that's the hook: Science finds the brain a world of wonderment. At the same time, a huge amount of other (non-stroke) brain science research is going on. This research, into   the brain and into recovery from brain injury, will rapidly continue to provide new insights. In the meantime, the extent to which the brain is able to rewire is not yet known. What we do know is that every time the brain is asked to do extraordinary things, it responds. That's the good news. The bad news is that the response takes a tremendous amount of hard work. This book celebrates and gives the scientific justification for that hard work.

THE SUPER-SURVIVOR

Every stroke survivor has a certain level of potential recovery. Few reach that potential. Stroke survivors who *do* reach their potential do so because they have no choice. This breed of "super-survivor" is so unwilling to let go of career independence, personal passions, family commitments, and so on, that they are compelled to recover. They intertwine recovery with what they love to do. Sometimes recovery is so much a part of what they love doing that they don't even notice they're recovering.

For the super-survivor, recovery is a vision quest. The challenge of recovery is no different from other challenges they've conquered in life. They get on with it. They put in the time. They fall in love with the process. It's much the same reason athletes, dancers, and muscians are driven to always get better. Stroke survivors who recover the most see the process of recovery as an opportunity for growth.

This book is not for stroke survivors who are okay with where they are. This is a book for stroke survivors who want to *get better*.

If you are not a stroke survivor, this book may have meaning for you as well. The same thing that drives recovery from stroke can drive any form of learning. Learning involves the most important scientific discovery since fire: *neuroplasticity*. Humans have always used their plastic brain. But the discovery of *how* the brain changes allows us to wonder: How much more can we make it change? How plastic is it? Answering these questions will help develop the best ways to recover from stroke. It will also help anyone trying to learn any new skill.

NEUROPLASTICITY AND HOW
SCIENCE GOT IT WRONG

In the mid-1800s, scientists began mapping the brain. Each portion of the brain was sectioned off. Each section was proclaimed as the *only* possible site for everything—from the ability to do math to wiggling your toes. One section, on the left side of the brain, always controls speech. Another section, near the top of the brain, controls the hand. The back of the brain processes vision; the front solves problems. These early attempts defined the brain as static. Sure, in our youth, perhaps before five years old, there were some changes in the brain. But after that initial wiring the brain was fixed, frozen, and locked. This was bad news for stroke survivors. What happened if the stroke killed the language portion of the brain? Because science thought the brain unchangeable, attempting to use different parts of the brain for language was, well ... *unthinkable*. Once language, or limb movement, or sensation, or anything else was knocked out by the stroke, it was gone. *Forever*.

There is good news, however: *These early attempts to define the brain were wrong.*

Scientists had a "mechanistic view" of the brain. Galileo and Copernicus had mechanized the heavens and Leonardo da Vinci had mechanized pretty much everything else. Our fascination with machines profoundly influenced our study of the human body. Scientists viewed the body as a machine, with smaller machines inside. Muscles were pulleys, bones were levers, the kidneys were filters, the heart was a pump, and so on. Certainly the brain was some sort of machine as well. Scientists tended to compare the brain to whatever the latest technology was: "The brain is like a clock." "The brain is like an engine." "The brain is like a calculator." Whatever the latest technology was, that's what the brain was like.

And then, in the mid-1900s, scientists started to realize that the brain did not operate like any other machine. Consider computers. If you ask two identical computers to do the same thing, they'll do the same thing in exactly the same way over and over and over again. But if you asked the same person the same question, once on Monday and once on Wednesday, they may very well give you different answers. They've "changed their mind." That change was actually a physical, measurable change in the brain. Neurons change structure and/or function.

Most of the work challenging the idea that "the brain is just another machine" came from neuroscience. Neuroscience studies the entire nervous system but is fascinated with the brain. Neuroscientists are especially interested in developing and testing ways of rewiring the brain neuroplastically. And this is good for folks that have brain injury, including stroke. Neuroplasticity is at the core of recovery. Neuroscience will lead the way in developing systems to drive neuroplasticity.

The ability the brain has to change, the ability to learn, comes at a cost. Our brain is inconsistent. A computer might always express A = B = C. We might say "A = C but I left out B because I'm in the process of adding D." As neuroscientists Sam Wang and Sandra Aamodt put it, the brain is less like machine and more like a busy Chinese restaurant. If you've ever been in a crowded Chinese restaurant, it's chaos. Some people are getting their orders taken, other people are being seated, orders are being yelled, food is being eaten, and plates are clanging.

But everything gets done.

Your brain is less like a computer and more like a busy Chinese restaurant. As new connections between neurons are made in the brain, different answers, different perspectives, and different solutions to problems are created. What we lose in the linear (A always = B, which always = C) we gain in the ability to do what other machines can't: *Learn*. And that's the point: Brains change, machines don't. As you read this book you may associate exercise with neurons and neurons with recovery and recovery with your own personal story. The brain can associate anything with anything else. Machines can only associate what you tell them to associate. Simply, brains learn, machines don't.

NEUROPLASTICITY: SIMPLICITY IN A BOX

The brain can be rewired and, under certain conditions, radically rearranged. It turns out that the brain, 100 billion neurons strong, can be changed into whatever kind of tool we want. And there is more good news: Some of the best tools needed for rewiring the brain after stroke are very simple. Although the brain is the most complex entity in the known universe, it responds and rewires according to simple instructions. All a person needs to change his or her brain is a whole lot of focused and dedicated practice. And it happens *fast*.

Large portions of our brains can be rewired in a matter of hours, days, or weeks. Understand: This is not some sort of vague "new-age" concept; this is an actual physical event, measurable by brain-scanning technology. From learning to control emotions to hitting a baseball, the core of change involves rewiring the brain.

You might suspect that there is a bit more to it, and there is. While the idea of "practice makes perfect" is simple, how to practice is more complicated. This book defines the elements needed to drive neuroplastic change.

Beyond focused and dedicated practice, rewiring the brain also involves another rather large pink elephant in the room: motivation. Neuroplasticity takes a tremendous amount of work. It does not necessarily involve a long period of time, just a lot of focused effort. Your hard work is the most essential aspect of successful recovery. Clearly, the most important person involved in the recovery from stroke is the survivor. Much of the work can be done at home with help from family and friends while under the guidance of doctors and therapists. While clinicians are essential to the recovery process, you and your caregivers should not wait for health professionals to chaperon you toward your highest level of potential recovery. There is no doctor, therapist, minister, guru, or shaman in a better position to run your master recovery plan. There is no one who cares as much. Accept the challenge, empower yourself, focus on recovery, work hard, don't give up, and watch an upward spiral emerge that allows for the highest level of recovery.

Introduction

We are what we repeatedly do.

—Aristotle

In the last decade or so, stroke-recovery research has focused on a few basic core concepts. Understanding these building blocks of recovery will help you decide which of the growing number of treatment options is right for you. All of the following will provide insight into developing a great recovery plan.

ELEMENTS ESSENTIAL TO RECOVERY FROM STROKE

Mixing the following elements has been shown to the drive neuroplastic (brain rewiring) change necessary for recovery:

Repetitive. Pick options that use repetitive practice. Movements that you want to relearn should be performed over and over. For instance, if you want to lift your foot better, then you would concentrate on doing that movement repeatedly and with the highest possible quality of movement. Use of repetition requires "nipping at the edges" of your current ability. With each attempt, try to extend beyond your present ability a little bit more. Repetitive practice changes the part of the brain that controls movement. But how many repetitions are needed to change the brain? Let's consider elbow extension (going from the elbow bent to the elbow straight). Approximately 1,200 repetitions are needed to make the brain better at controlling that movement. Not perfect, but better. And that's for a single-joint movement.

Most of the movements we make involve many joints moving in a variety of directions. So how many repetitions are needed to do complex "every day" movements? The number of repetitions needed gets very large very quickly. Most practical everyday movements will require tens of thousands, if not hundreds of thousands, of repetitions. This is one of the reasons that working only when a therapist is around is not practical. There is simply not enough time with therapists to accomplish the number of repetitions needed.

New and Challenging. Work on movements that are novel (new) to you. Of course, the movements are not really new. You may have been doing the movements for 50 years prior to your stroke, but it is considered novel if it has yet to be learned since your stroke. Researchers use the word "novel," but a better word may be "challenging." Focus on relearning challenging movements. Attempting movements that are too easy will not help you recover. As soon as you can perform a movement at a quality that reaches about 80 percent of your pre-stroke ability, move on to something new and challenging.

Meaningful. Neuroplastic (brain rewiring) change is much more likely to occur if the movement you are trying to relearn is part of a real-world task. The task has to be meaningful (important, essential, engaging) to you. The more important the task is to you, the more it will drive recovery. For instance, if you are trying to regain the ability to pick up objects, make it part of a real-world task that is meaningful to you.

Use what you care about to drive recovery. Recover to do what you care about.

If you love to paint, practice picking up a paintbrush. But what if you can't pick up a paintbrush? You only need to practice a portion of the task. It is not necessary to have the ability to accomplish the entire task to make it task specific. If the task is picking up a paintbrush, you may only be able to get the hand to the table but not be able to actually grasp the brush. As you bring the hand up to the table, have the paintbrush there to provide a meaningful goal.

THE P.E.N.S. CONCEPT

The P.E.N.S. concept provides an effective way to decide whether or not an option is worthy of consideration. It includes:

P is for *Patient driven*.

- Can you do the therapy by yourself, or does it require supervision?

- Is it intuitive, or does it require a lot of training? Is it expensive or is it affordable?

- Is it available in your area or do you have to travel to get to it?

Lean toward options that have the potential to be used at home, relatively easily, and with little cost and set-up.

E is for *Evidence based*. Has the option been researched? The amount of scientific testing of recovery options is highly variable. Some …

- Have never been tested

- Have been tested in small, poorly run studies

- Have been tested by people who will make money if the product sells

- Have done poorly in well-run studies

- Have done poorly in multiple well-run studies

- Have done well in well-run studies

- Have done well in multiple well-run studies

When researching the recovery option, ask the question: Did it shine or was it a lemon? In the Resources section of this book there are websites and other sources of information to help you pick and choose.

N is for *Neuroplastic*. Does the recovery option promote neuroplastic change? That is, will it rewire the brain in a way that helps recovery? The problem is, science may not have yet proven that the option you've chosen actually rewires the brain. There are few recovery options that have been tested this way. Try to determine if the therapy has all the earmarks of neuroplasticity included in Essential Elements of Recovery From Stroke, discussed previously.

S is for *Simulations* vectors. This is a fancy way of saying, "Consider multiple options as you plan your recovery." There is no one magic bullet for stroke recovery. Therapists tend to use a small group of therapies that they know well. Researchers tend to focus on a small group of related treatment options. Both therapists and researchers bring important perspectives to stroke recovery.

But in some ways, both lack a sufficiently broad perspective. When stroke recovery is viewed globally, a hidden secret emerges: It's not anything, it's everything. Imagine stroke recovery as a picture puzzle. Solving the stroke-recovery puzzle involves using the puzzle pieces (recovery options) to build as complete a picture as possible (recovery). If the puzzle is done correctly, the highest possible level of recovery is achieved. The stroke-recovery puzzle has two added dimensions that picture puzzles don't:

1. The number of pieces (treatment options) is continually changing. This is a result of increased research, including research of new technologies. At the same time, research is sifting out other, ineffective treatments.

2. The background picture (where you are in the recovery arc) changes.

Figuring out . . .

- what puzzle piece fits
- when it fits
- and how it fits

. . . is essential to an effective recovery plan.

GOOD NEWS AND BAD NEWS

Recovery takes hard work and commitment. It's not easy. It will most likely be the hardest thing you've ever done. But the *process* is simple.

- The bad news: Recovery takes a lot of hard work.
  Note: If someone is telling you that they can help you recover without hard work, grab your wallet and leave!

- The good news: The process of recovering from stroke is both intuitive and simple.
  Note: If someone is telling you to do something to recover but they can't explain why in simple language—it is cause for suspicion!

ONE LAST BIT OF HOUSEKEEPING . . .

While limbs on one side of the body are most impacted, research has found that all four limbs are affected by the brain damage caused by stroke.

Because all four limbs are affected, researchers use the terms "more affected" and "less affected" when describing the relative deficit in the limbs after stroke. Please note that for the sake of brevity and simplicity, this book sometimes uses the following terms:

- "Bad"—the limbs more affected by the stroke.
- "Good"—the limbs less affected by the stroke.

These terms are not meant to reflect the potential for recovery, nor the relative importance of the limb.

Acknowledgments

I would like to thank:

All the stroke survivors and caregivers I've communicated with over the past two decades. Successful survivors hold the key to recovery.

My wife, Aila Mella, who has had a profound influence on this book. Aila was one of my clinical instructors back in school and has continued to teach me through the many, many conversations we've had about stroke recovery and rehabilitation.

Dr. Stephen J. Page, my friend and colleague, who helped forge my perspective on stroke recovery and has provided the tools and support to everyone in our lab who has worked toward developing novel ways to helps survivors recover. Steve has been our lab's fearless leader from the early days at the Kessler Institute, through the early 2000s at University of Cincinnati, right up to the present at The Ohio State University.

The members of the Kessler Rehabilitation's Human Performance Movement Analysis Lab, for teaching me the nuts and bolts of clinical research.

The scientists that helped all of us "connect the dots" between the many branches of science and stroke recovery, including **Karl Lashley, Vilayanur S. Ramachandran**, and **Alvaro Pascual-Leone**. Special thanks to **Signe Brunnström, Edward Taub, Michelle Ploughman**, and **Jeffrey Kleim**, for laying bare the connection among neuroscience, psychology, and the therapeutic interventions that drive recovery.

Occupational therapist Aimee Fay for helping me understand the impact of psychosocial problems after stroke on physical recovery.

My mom, Rosemarye Massa Levine, and dad, Martin Levine, for encouraging and supporting me during all of my education.

My children, Emma Maria Levine and Jesse Martin Levine, because work is best done when it is balanced with what children bring: *Fun!*

Stronger After Stroke

1 Stroke Recovery Essentials

PLAN YOUR WORK AND WORK YOUR PLAN

Every great journey starts with a great plan. An ambitious recovery plan is vital to your recovery. The plan begins to evolve in the hospital, right after the stroke, and it continues to develop during your time in:

- Skilled nursing facilities
- Rehabilitation hospitals
- Outpatient clinics
- Home therapy

The early portion of the plan is easy because therapists are developing and implementing the plan. What do you do after occupational, physical, and speech therapies have ended? Stroke survivors typically face the rest of their lives, and the rest of the struggle toward recovery, with no formal recovery plan. Once the standard therapies have ended, the power of your plan becomes even more vital. This is a critical time in recovery. There are three options you can choose from:

1. You believe that, because your therapy has ended, your recovery has ended.

2. You are willing to continue your recovery, but you are not sure what to work on. You decide that you'll join a gym and see what happens.

3. You develop a plan that takes you to the highest level of recovery possible. You know that your plan will change over time. Your plan has built-in goals. Achieving goals gives rise to new goals and new achievements. This forces an upward spiral of recovery.

How Is It Done?

A powerful and successful recovery plan will:

- *Be measurable*: The recovery plan includes specific goals and land-marks that represent breakthroughs in the recovery process. These breakthroughs are predicted by the plan. The same way coaches set goals for athletes, your plan should set goals that promote recovery. Examples of measurable goals include:
  - — "I will be able to walk fifty yards at my daughter's wedding in three months."
  - — "I will be able to use a fork and knife by Christmas."
  - — "I will be able to pull rope, hand over hand, on my sailboat by next summer."
- *Be flexible*: Stroke recovery involves a constantly shifting set of opportunities. The choice of recovery options and exercises that you'll use will change as you recover. A flexible recovery plan allows for quick adjustments to promote further recovery. For instance, consider the goal, "I will be able to pick up a cup with my bad hand." Once you are able to do this, the plan is adjusted to provide a new challenge (e.g., "I will be able to pick up and drink from a cup"). The goal is made more difficult to promote even more recovery.
- *Encourage self-reliance*: Focus on recovery techniques that you under-stand and can carry out yourself. When you can perform the recovery technique without the aid of a clinician, you provide yourself with more opportunity to recover. Promoting self-reliance allows you to recover even after formal therapies have ended. This do-it-yourself spin on recovery allows you to take control of the process.
- *Include short- and long-term goals*: A short-term goal is to walk ten feet. A long-term goal is to walk without a limp. The long-term goal is made with the series of short-term goals in mind. As a metaphor, the long-term goals are the blueprints for a house made of brick. The short-term goals are bricks.

What Precautions Should Be Taken?

Any plan should be done within parameters of safety. Consider the examples, "I will be able to walk a quarter mile in ten minutes, and I will accomplish this by Christmas." Walking long distances has obvious inherent risks. On the other hand, a goal like, "I will be able to open my hand enough to grasp a cup handle within the next month" may rely simply on repetitions of opening and closing the hand, and so contains little risk. "Safety first" is essential to the recovery process, because nothing stops recovery like an injury.

SAY NO TO PLATEAU

Therapists will stop treating you when they can no longer measure improvement. This lack of progress toward recovery is commonly called a plateau. Plateau means "flattening out." If you have "plateaued" it means that, according to clinicians, you are not getting any better. If it is determined that a survivor has plateaued, most insurance coverage ends. From the survivor's point of view, the act of ending treatment too often says "That's it. You won't get any better." In many stroke survivors, this has an unfortunate dual effect. First, the end of therapy means the end of the support, guidance, and expertise of therapists. Second, saying that a stroke survivor is no longer making progress often (but thankfully not always) becomes a self-fulfilling prophecy. The stroke survivor thinks, "The professionals who know the most about stroke recovery believe that I'm not going to get any better. I guess that's all I can expect." This assumption is not correct. There are several reasons for mistaken assumptions about when recovery has ended.

- Some healthcare professionals suggest that during the **chronic** phase of stroke (usually defined as starting three months after stroke), no further recovery can be made. The truth is that stroke survivors can continue to make progress years, even decades, after their stroke.

- A process known as learned nonuse (described fully in the section Constraint-Induced Therapy for the Arm and Hand in Chapter 4) may have taken place during the subacute phase. Learned nonuse is reversible, even during the chronic phase.

- To save money, payers (insurance, Medicare, etc.) put pressure on therapists to end therapy as soon as possible. Therapists would prefer to treat stroke survivors for longer periods, but they cannot. The result is that therapy is usually ended before the fullest possible recovery is realized.

- The tests that therapists use are often not sensitive enough to detect small but important changes in recovery. For instance, tests of spasticity and reflexes can indicate progress toward recovery, but these two tests are rarely done in therapy settings. Other tests that are "stroke specific" (tests that are used only for stroke) are usually not done. These tests can detect small but important advances in recovery. So the question is: Is there really no progress, or are the wrong tests being used?

- Simply, your recovery could progress, but the most effective recovery options are not used. Clinically, these options may not be used for one of the following reasons:

  — Lack of therapist training in the new therapy

  — Lack of support for the therapy by the rehabilitation facility

  — Payers do not pay for the therapy

  — Clinicians are unaware of the therapy

  — The therapy does not make a profit

- Survivors and their families often push for release from the rehab facilities as soon as possible. Therapists are sensitive to this. Therapists work to help patients get as safe and as functional as quickly as possible. Rushing the survivor through the system means:

  — Less time is spent recovering

  — Less guidance is available

  — Less recovery is attained

- Therapists focus on helping you become functional and safe. **Functional** is defined as the ability to do useful or practical activities. For instance, if you can dress yourself, even if you don't use your "bad" arm and hand, you are considered functional in dressing. Walking safely, even if it involves a cane and orthosis on your foot, is considered functional walking. Being functional will get you home and help you get on with your life. But being functional does not usually represent the highest possible level of recovery you can achieve.

Achieving the highest possible level of recovery requires extending beyond functional ability.

The word **plateau** has been used by clinicians to describe the point at which "no further recovery can be made." But not everyone considers a plateau a negative thing. Athletes have used the word for decades. A plateau to an athlete is different from the way plateau is used to describe the end of recovery after stroke. Athletes define a plateau as a point in their training where their present training techniques no longer help them get better, stronger, or faster. Athletes respond to a plateau by trying new strategies to improve their ability. Stroke survivors should view a plateau the same way athletes do—as an opportunity to re-evaluate and modify the recovery plan.

How Is It Done?

Many of the suggestions in this book can help you overcome temporary plateaus. But the most important suggestion is this: Assume that there will be no lasting plateau. Assuming no limits to recovery may be optimistic, but it allows for the largest opportunity for the highest level of recovery. If you want to get better, assume you will return to the same level of ability you enjoyed prior to the stroke. You may not achieve full recovery, but you'll still have extended further than the supposed plateau.

If your recovery efforts are not producing results, a temporary plateau will follow. When this happens, and it will, do what athletes do and change your training techniques. Athletes look at it this way: "I've been using training technique 'X', and it's been great. 'X' got me this far. But now I've plateaued. If I continue with 'X,' the plateau will continue. But if I change my training, I may be able to achieve a new, higher plateau." Survivors can look at it the same way. The same strategies will yield the same results. New strategies will yield new results. Challenge your **physiatrist** and therapists with suggestions of techniques, treatments, and technologies that you find during your research. If you see something that you think might work, ask these clinicians to use them. Remember: Therapy was most likely stopped because these health professionals believed that recovery ended. If therapists just continued to use the same techniques, then, indeed, you would not improve further. The same techniques will likely generate the same results. In your own attempts toward recovery, look for new recovery options that might work.

There is another benefit to exceeding a plateau on your own: Progress can be used to justify more funding for therapy. Remember, discharge from therapy happened because no progress was being made. If you can show that progress has been made—on your own, since the discharge—insurance will view this change in status as a trigger for more therapy.

What Precautions Should Be Taken?

There are some instances where stroke survivors cannot achieve any more movement than they have at a given point in time. This is usually the case only when the stroke survivor does not have the mental capacity to try.

USE YOUR FANTASTIC PLASTIC BRAIN

Here are a couple of "mind blowers": The human brain is the most complex structure in the universe. There are approximately 100 billion neurons (nerve cells) in the brain.

But that number is small compared to the number of connections between neurons in the brain. The present estimate of connections between neurons is an astounding quadrillion (a thousand trillion). But that vast number is not set in stone at birth; the number of connections can be radically increased. Anyone can increase connections at any time throughout their life, well into old age. This is usually done by learning something substantial and new.

Recovery from stroke often involves increasing the number and quality of these connections in the brain. Increasing the number of connections is determined by the hard work of the survivor. Forging new connections between the neurons that survive the stroke is the basis for much of the recovery from stroke.

Recovery will naturally follow from working with the one organ damaged by the stroke and from which all true recovery comes: *the brain*. In order to recover, stroke survivors have to rewire their brains. The technical term is **neuroplasticity**.

Neuroplasticity is a long word that, like so many medical words, can be broken down to determine the meaning. "Neuro" basically means having to do with nerves. The second half of the word is *plasticity* (from the Latin *plasticus*, which means *molding*). The root word is *plastic*. Plastic, when it is heated, becomes flexible and can be molded into almost any shape. Neuroplasticity allows the brain, within limits, to be quickly and massively remolded.

Neuroplastic change happens in all of us, all the time, and happens without us knowing a neuron from a necktie. Harnessing and directing the power of plasticity is the focus of most of modern stroke-specific rehabilitation research.

One of the proven ways to rewire the brain is called **repetitive practice**. Repetitive practice involves repeatedly practicing a movement, even if you can only do a small part of that movement.

One of the things that stroke survivors often ask is, "How many times do I have to attempt a movement before I see improvement?" Or, "How many repetitions do I have to do before I rewire my brain?" Survivors and therapists will often ask the "How many?" question of researchers that work in rehabilitation research. Therapists have a good reason for wanting to know this number: They have limited time with the survivor before they discharge the survivor from therapy. So knowing a specific number of repetitions helps the therapist know the number of repetitions—per session—that the survivor would have to do to recover.

For a long time, those of us in research didn't know the answer. We would say things like "A lot," and "As many as you can do." The problem was, we only had good data for people who had learned how to move really well. Included would be professional musicians, cigar rollers in Cuba, carpet weavers in Iran, and college and professional athletes. How many repetitions do those people need? To become a high-level expert at something (e.g., a professional basketball player, carpet weaver, or musician), the number of repetitions needed are in the millions. You cannot tell a therapist that they should have survivors do millions of repetitions. The therapist will look at you cock-eyed and (sometimes politely) ask. "Do you know where I work? Sometimes I have problems getting survivors out of bed!"

But then we were saved! There is a certain breed of therapist that goes back to school and gets a PhD in neuroscience—the branch of science that studies the brain. These therapists have one foot back in the clinic (they are often therapists at heart). And because of their doctorate in neuroscience, they know a lot about the brain. And these therapists have done experiments to try to figure out the "How many repetitions are needed to recover?" question. These researchers will scan the brain and measure movement as the survivor adds more repetitions. So what did they find out? How many repetitions do survivors need?

Let's put it this way: There is some good news and some bad news (and some more good news):

Good news:

The number of repetitions needed for a survivor to get better movement at one joint: approximately 1,200. Note that the actual number will be different for every survivor. The 1,200 number is the average,

Bad news:

The average number of repetitions a survivor does during an hour-long session with a therapist: is 25 to 35.

More good news:

Studies have shown that if the therapist and survivor focus only on repetitive movements during an hour-long session, the numbers can get real high real fast—in the 300 to 500 range. Survivors, working on their own, within the limits of safety, can reach very high numbers as well.

But there is a bit more bad news. Computing the number for stroke survivors is tricky. Let's consider the "1,200" number. That number was found to be true for one movement at one joint. That is, in order to change the brain enough to make just one movement better, you would need 1,200 repetitions. Consider **dorsiflexion** (lifting the foot at the ankle). This movement is essential for walking. In order to gain more dorsiflexion, a survivor would need to do (approximately) at least 1,200 repetitions. But that's just for that one movement at that one joint. Walking involves many movements at many joints (technically known as "multi-joint, multiplanar movement"). And all the other joints— besides dorsiflexion—in all the other planes (directions) would also have to be practiced repeatedly. This is why the number of repetitions for most functional movement (like walking, dressing, eating) is both *large* and *difficult* to estimate.

- **The number of repetitions is large** because many joints move in many directions in order to do common tasks.

- **The estimation of the number of repetitions is difficult** because the number of repetitions would be "survivor specific." That is, every survivor, given their unique deficits, would require a different number of repetitions.

The number varies for each survivor depending on:

- The complexity of the movement to be relearned
- The amount of movement currently available
- The intensity and focus with which the repetitions are done
- The age of the survivor
- The health of the survivor besides the stroke
- And so on (the list of variables that can impact the number of repetitions needed is long)

How Is It Done?

You are the only person who can rewire your brain. The best therapist in the world can't do it for you. Neuroplasticity, and the recovery that results, emerges from the inside out. The more focused repetitions of a movement the more the brain has a chance to rewire, reconfigure, and rebuild.

Neuroplasticity happens fast. There are classic scientific experiments that prove that large portions of the brain can be rewired with little more than four days of dedicated work. There is a catch, however. Rewiring the brain after stroke requires hard and focused work. Some stroke survivors may not have the cognitive ability or the mental focus required to rewire their brains using neuroplasticity. This is the case only if the stroke survivor has lost the ability to *try*.

Neuroplastic change happens to all of us, all the time. The smallest event—from humming a tune to catching a set of keys—will cause neuroplastic change. However, if a skill is developed with the right intensity, it will promote lasting change in the brain. The saying among scientists who examine how the brain works is "neurons that fire together wire together." Here is how this concept works. Imagine you are standing on the beach, ten feet from the water's edge. You have a bucket of water, and you pour the water toward the ocean. You pour the first bucket of water. It flows a few inches and then becomes absorbed by the sand. The second bucket travels a foot or two. The third bucket extends even farther. After a few more buckets of water, you have formed a creek to the ocean. All the water that you pour then flows easily to the sea. Neurons (nerve cells) in the brain work much the same way. Every time you move, you forge new connections to make that movement easier and easier until you can perform the movement without thinking. Neuroplastic change is the result of the same set of neurons in the brain firing, over and over, in the same way.

The process needed to rewire your brain does not need to be fully understood to benefit from its power. Simply, the brain can be treated like a "black box." If you put in the right kind of focused, repetitive effort, you get out better movement. It is the movement of different parts of your body that rewires the brain. That is, actively moving your limbs, mouth, trunk, and so forth, will rewire the brain. In this way, movement of the body rewires the brain, and rewiring the brain makes movement better. A virtuous circle!

How do you know your repetitive practice is working? Increased coordination will be the proof positive that your brain is being rewired. This is why accurately measuring progress by testing the amount and quality of movement is so important. If there is neuroplastic change, that change will produce better movement. The better the movement, the more the brain has rewired.

Neuroplasticity is something that musicians and athletes use all the time. And the way musicians, athletes, and stroke survivors access neuroplasticity is exactly the same: focused practice. The same efforts that help athletes and musicians become the best they can be can help stroke survivors rewire their brains to navigate around the area of brain tissue killed by the stroke. If enough of this rewiring occurs, the stroke survivor can make progress, even when in the chronic phase (sometimes defined as more than three months after stroke) of recovery. Scientists, with the aid of brain scanning technology, have proven that the brain can rewire. Other tests including kinematics, kinetics, **electromyography**, and other outcome measures have been used as well. All of these tests have shown a direct link between brain rewiring and improved movement and function.

The trick to rewiring the brain after stroke is finding recovery options that promote neuroplastic change. The tools that rewire the brain range from highly sophisticated robots (i.e., recovery machines; see Chapter 9) to simple repetitive and demanding practice. Other brain rewiring strategies outlined in this book include:

- Bilateral training (see the section titled The Good Trains the Bad—Bilateral Training in Chapter 4)

- Constraint-induced therapy (CIT; see the section in Chapter 4 titled Constraint-Induced Therapy for the Arm and Hand)

- Mental practice (see Chapter 4, the Imagine It! section) will drive rewiring of the brain

- Electrical stimulation (see the section Get Your Hand Back in Chapter 4)

- Mirror therapy (see Chapter 4, the section on Mirror Therapy)

What Precautions Should Be Taken?

The level of commitment needed to rewire your brain requires the guidance of your doctors, nurses, and therapists. Safety is essential. Many of the concepts in this book ask for an increased amount of time, effort, and repetitions of movements. These efforts, in turn, require increased muscle, heart, and lung effort. Neuroplasticity is fatiguing because it is a physical process in the brain. Bluntly, learning to move better after stroke—called **motor learning**—is fatiguing. But rewiring the brain also involves working weak muscles. So rewiring the brain involves fatigue from both building your muscles and changing your brain. Fatigue can lead to unsafe efforts and unsafe decision making. Be careful as you change your fantastic plastic brain.

A DOCTOR MADE FOR STROKE SURVIVORS

There are many types of doctors that can help folks that have had stroke—from neurologists to primary care physicians. But there is one kind of medical doctor who has specific training in stroke recovery: **physiatrists** (fizz-EYE-uh trists). Their medical training and special knowledge of stroke recovery make physiatrists vital to the process of recovery.

Physiatrists are often called "stroke doctors" because they are the medical professionals that patients most often associate with treatment for impairments caused by stroke. Physiatrists:

- Know the latest stroke-related medical treatments and will be able to prescribe the most appropriate medications
- Do special testing that will help determine where you are in recovery
- Are able to design a recovery plan that focuses on the medical side of recovery, including spasticity reduction and pain control
- Have a large number of tools at their disposal to help foster the continuation of recovery from stroke

How Is It Done?

After their therapy ends, most stroke survivors never visit a physiatrist again. In fact, most stroke survivors don't even remember what a physiatrist is a few years past their stroke. Because of this lost relationship, survivors are unaware of years of medical advancements that can impact their recovery. I even have a joke about it: *When a stroke survivor is asked, a couple of years after his stroke, who his physiatrist is, he says, "There's nothing wrong with my feet!"*

Ask your primary care physician for a referral to a physiatrist. Get recommendations from other stroke survivors. Look for an aggressive physiatrist who is willing to work with you as you actively strive toward full recovery. Visiting a physiatrist can help set up an upward spiral in your recovery. For instance:

- You visit a physiatrist.
- The physiatrist treats your spasticity.
- Since your spasticity has reduced, the physiatrist writes a prescription for therapy to help build on movements unmasked by your newly loosened muscles. A visit to a physiatrist will often trigger a prescription for more therapy.
- The reduction in spasticity combined with therapy leads to recovery of lost movement.
- Recovery of lost movement allows you to challenge yourself with other new movements.

There are several other reasons to see a physiatrist that may or may not be directly related to recovery from stroke. The following should automatically trigger a visit to a physiatrist:

- Pain that limits the ability to move or function
- Spasticity that makes a limb hard to move
- Falls
- Loss of normal bowel and bladder function

What Precautions Should Be Taken?

When talking to a physiatrist, listen to everything suggested, but also guide the doctor toward what you specifically want to accomplish. For instance, saying, "I want to be able to open my hand" is more effective than "I want to move better."

NEUROSCIENCE: YOUR NEW BEST FRIEND

The last couple of decades have produced an explosion in our understanding of stroke recovery. Because of the overwhelming interest in the brain (stroke *is* brain injury), many branches of science have lent their skill and energy to the question of stroke recovery. From exercise physiology to psychology, from electronics to genetics, interest in stroke recovery has radically broadened. But of all the branches of science that have lent their voices to this discussion, one has had the most impact: neuroscience. Neuroscience is very interested in brain plasticity. The ability for the brain to remake itself is the focus of much of neuroscience. Everyone has a brain, but we're not sure of the best ways to change it. Finding the best ways to change it is what neuroscience aims to do. Neuroplasticity (the ability for the brain to rewire according to the will of its owner) can be defined in another, much simpler word: *learning*. So neuroscientists are interested in learning. And learning to move after stroke (called **motor learning**) is interesting to neuroscientists because it provides a unique window to *all* learning.

Stroke survivors often lose a part of the brain that controls movement. Stroke survivors can be tested to determine which recovery strategies help survivors move better. But there is a problem. Just because science says something works doesn't mean that it will be used. Researchers call this "a lack of transition from benchside to bedside." Researchers lament that what research reveals "benchside" (in laboratories) is not necessarily being used "bedside" (treatments that stroke survivors are actually receiving).

Science is still discovering the extent to which the brain can rewire. But there *is* one thing we're sure of. *Given the right circumstances, the brain can radically rewire over a very short period of time.* What science has learned about the plasticity of the brain is good news for stroke survivors. Despite all we've learned, however, clinicians treating stroke survivors don't necessarily view stroke recovery as having anything to do with the brain. Since clinicians can't typically see the brain rewiring, they focus on what they *can* see. Clinicians usually look at stroke patients in terms of "functional ability" (ability to do everyday tasks). Typically, the goal of stroke rehabilitation is simple: Get survivors as functional as possible, and get them "home" as soon as possible. This focus on function is not just practical, it's what managed care (insurance) is willing to pay for.

There is a downside to this focus on function, however. Function does not equal recovery. For instance, a survivor could put on his shirt and pants without moving his affected arm at all. Function does not necessarily reflect what's going on in the brain.

Consider this thought experiment. "Tom," a survivor, had his stroke six weeks ago. He is in a rehabilitation hospital getting therapy from great therapists. However, the therapists have noted a "stalling" of his progress. His occupational and physical therapists agree: Tom is making little progress.

Typically, if a patient has stalled in their recovery (called a **plateau**) the patient is discharged. Since Tom is no longer making progress, therapy must end. The thinking is, if no progress is being made, why should more money be spent?

Now, let's say Tom's brain is *right at the beginning* of the brain rewiring (neuroplastic) process. The beginning of the rewiring process reveals itself in small amounts of movement. In fact, the small increases may be real, but clinicians do not often measure these small changes. These small but important changes are not measured for two reasons:

1. Therapists do not have the tools (called outcome measures) that are sensitive enough to pick up these small but important changes.

2. Small amounts of movement are considered "nonfunctional"; that is, clinicians may observe new movement but since the movement does not lead to function (walking, dressing, eating) it is considered ... *unimportant*.

But small amounts of movement, while not yet providing function, are essential to the incremental process of recovery. Unfortunately, therapy may instead focus on using the "good side" to help the patient regain more function. Thus, the focus on function is really a focus on the "good side." Because of this focus on function the part of the brain that controls the "good side" (ironically) rewires a lot. That's where the focus is, so that's what rewires. At the same time, the part of the brain that controls the "bad side" doesn't rewire because nothing is being asked of it. This process is at the core of **learned nonuse** (described fully in the section in Chapter 4 titled Constraint-Induced Therapy for the Arm and Hand).

In the typical rehab setting, function is not only the goal, it's what's tested. Typically, these tests will focus on "activities of daily living" (ADLs) like walking, dressing, toileting. These tests are not very nuanced. The survivor can either walk, dress, or toilet, or they can't. The only nuance is trying to determine the amount of assistance needed to do the task. The assistance needed involves four broad categories.

Levels of Functional Ability

- Independent: No assistance is needed.
- Minimum assistance needed: The survivor needs the caregiver to help with less than 25 percent of the effort needed to accomplish that function.

- Moderate assistance needed: The caregiver provides 25 to 50 percent of effort.

- Maxlmal asslstance needed: The caregiver provides 50 to 75 percent of effort.

Once survivors have reached their highest level of functional ability they are discharged from therapy (therapy is ended). "The highest level of functional ability" is called the *plateau*, an assumed endpoint of recovery.

But neuroscience is challenging this concept by asking, "Are these really limitations imposed by the brain, or are these limits caused by the nature of rehabilitation treatment and tests?" Here's another way of asking this question: "Are survivors treated according to convention or science?" These questions have become the foundation of a new perspective on stroke recovery, and, again, neuroscience is the vanguard of this new perspective. Neuroscientists view recovery not in terms of function, but in terms of the function of the brain. Because they focus on the brain, they tend to be much more optimistic about recovery from stroke than clinicians. In the average stroke (stress *average*), a small percentage of neurons (nerve cells) in the brain die. But because of the focus on function, that small number of neurons has a huge impact on the brain. Again, this process is known as **learned nonuse**. Stopping learned nonuse from asserting its influence on the brain is the most important goal of the subacute phase. Ideas for keeping the influence on learned nonuse to a minimum are discussed in Chapter 6 in the section The Subacute Phase: Recovery's Sweet Spot.

How Is It Done?

Neuroscience has radically changed the way stroke recovery is understood. Traditionally, stroke recovery research had been done by clinicians with a lot of clinical experience (experience treating patients). In other words, researchers who study stroke recovery don't start out as researchers. They start out as clinicians. Their experience in the clinic profoundly influences their research. Because they are typically "clinicians first" they often view survivors as vulnerable and frail patients. Their clinical experience tells them that most stroke survivors are older and have other diseases (heart problems, diabetes, orthopedic issues, etc.) as well as stroke. Their research is influenced by the perceived frailty of the body, not the plasticity of the brain.

Classic clinical research for stroke recovery has other problems as well. When you do research, you're looking for (as much as you can) a "one-size-fits-all" treatment. Consider the following statements:

- "Aspirin reduces pain."
- "Exercise reduces blood pressure."
- "Caffeine makes people more alert."

These statements have been proven true in healthy people. If you're doing research on healthy people, you can choose any healthy person to participate in your study. But what if you are studying stroke survivors? How do you find "the average stroke survivor"? *Every stroke is different.* This statement is true in so many ways. For instance, each stroke . . .

- Is unique in its size and shape
- Affects different parts of the brain
- Causes different deficits

Also, each stroke *survivor* . . .

- Is a specific age
- Has a unique level of motivation
- Has a different level of overall health
- Has different goals
- Has a different amount of time since the stroke

Because of this, clinicians in rehab research find it difficult to develop "one-size-fits-all" treatments. This is where neuroscience has a great advantage. Neuroscientists often work with animals. The animals they usually work with are rats or mice. Rats and mice are good for stroke recovery research for a number of reasons. They . . .

- Are inexpensive
- Are easy to work with (compared to other animals)
- Have hands that move in a very human-like way

Neuroscientists can intentionally give rats a stroke. They give rats strokes in a number of ways. One way is to surgically block an artery that feeds blood to the brain. Another way is to send a pulse of water into the rat's brain. Researchers do this by using a specialized funnel that goes through the skull. A pulse of water is sent into the funnel, through the skull, killing a very specific part of the brain. Also, neuroscientists can use groups of rats that are very similar in terms of age, diet, health, environment, upbringing, and so on. The end result is that you have a lot of very similar "patients" who have had very similar strokes.

Beyond having access to an animal population with very similar strokes, rats provide another advantage. Consider this question: We know that intensity (a whole lot of hard work) helps survivors recover. We also know too much too early after stroke can reduce recovery (during the **acute phase** the brain is too vulnerable). So here's the question: When should therapy get intensive, and how intensive should therapy get? In humans, this sort of research would be considered unethical for many reasons. Let's say researchers wanted to test very intensive therapy early after the stroke. We know that the brain is very vulnerable immediately after the stroke, so any survivor you have doing intensive therapy could suffer. Research that has the potential to hurt humans is unethical and illegal. In fact, the rules to do any kind of study of humans are very strict, and permission to do a human study is difficult to get. So, a study that has any potential to harm humans in any way would never see the light of day.

But researchers can do just about anything (within reason) with rats. They could do very intensive therapy with the rats soon after they wake up from their stroke. Researchers might force them to swim or run for long distances (with their "good" paws) right after their stroke. Rat brains can be scanned in the same way the human brain can be scanned. Also, their limbs can be tested for any movement gains (or losses).

Researchers can test other things with rats that would be unethical in humans. Consider what is called "an enriched environment." We're pretty sure that an enriched environment (lots of social interactions, things to play with, etc.) help stroke survivors recover. But to test this, some survivors would have the enriched environment and other survivors would be to be isolated in a room with no social interaction. This is clearly unethical in humans. But this sort of research has been done with rats. One group of rats is put in separate cages in separate rooms with nothing but food. A second group of rats is put with a lot of other rats and with a lot of toys to play with. The rats who are in the enriched environments after stroke recover more. This information, that "enrichment = recovery" can be used by clinicians and caregivers to help survivors recover.

And it's not just "enriched environments" that can be tested. Using a rat model, you could test just about any variable, including sleep, diet, exercise, environment, temperature, and so on.

How Neuroscience Can Help Stroke Survivors

What are the secrets that neuroscience has revealed? Here is a short list of some of the most remarkable insights neuroscience has provided.

- Behavior changes the brain. The brain rewires according to the survivor's behavior.

- Although estimates vary, the average human brain has approximately 100 billion neurons. The average stroke destroys just over 1 percent of those neurons (1.2 billion). Neuroscientists are asking: Why, in the highly plastic human brain, does such a small amount of damage (less than 2 percent) have such a devastating effect on the average survivor?

  — Neuroscience is beginning to understand how **learned nonuse**, and not just the amount of damage to the brain, determines the impact of the stroke. Learned nonuse is something that's controllable in the rehabilitation setting. That is, the way rehabilitation is provided may increase or decrease learned nonuse.

- Enriched environments (environments with a lot of social interactions and conversations, games, and things to "play" with) help the recovery of movement. Unfortunately, stroke decreases opportunities for social interaction.

  — In the first few weeks after stroke, survivors are alone approximately 60 percent of the time and they are inactive (resting or sitting) 75 percent of the time. Neuroscience research suggests that enriched environments during what is usually "downtime" promotes recovery.

  — Enriched environments are good for the brain after stroke. Enriched environments increase:

    – The number of branches (dendrites) produced by neurons (nerve cells in the brain)

    – The number of connections between neurons (synapses)

    – The number of cells that support neurons (called glial cells)

    – The number of blood vessels that deliver blood to the brain

— Enriched environments (interesting experiences, conversations, play, etc.) help recovery of movement. Unfortunately, stroke decreases opportunities to work within a complex environment.

- If done in the first ten days after stroke, focused training of the "good side" worsens future function of the "bad" side. Further, this negative effect extends to later efforts to rehabilitate the "good" side.

- Too much intensity of rehab in the first seven days after stroke can hurt function.

- When survivors exercise intensively (or "a lot") and voluntarily during the first seven days of stroke, brain plasticity is *decreased*.

- When survivors exercise intensively and voluntarily starting 14 to 20 days after stroke, brain plasticity is *increased*.

- There are specific windows of opportunity after stroke in which the brain is highly plastic (moldable).

    — In rat studies . . .

    - Therapy started between 5 and 14 days after stroke had the most recovery

    - Therapy started at 30 days after stroke had very little recovery

One more note about the neuroscience perspective on stroke recovery. There are many neuroscientists that are interested in the effect of a particular protein on brain rewiring. The protein is called **brain-derived neurotrophic factor**, or simply BDNF. BDNF has been called "Miracle Grow™ for the brain." It is produced in the brain, and supports learning. BDNF "primes" the brain for **motor learning**—the sort of learning that helps survivors recover movement. BDNF is produced naturally right after birth, which makes sense, because the brain must massively wire right after birth. It also is produced right after brain injuries, including stroke. This is one of the reasons that the subacute phase after stroke is so important. During the subacute phase, the brain is awash in BDNF. This is one of the reasons the subacute phase provides such unique opportunities for recovery. You will find ideas for getting the most out of the subacute phase in The Subacute Phase: Recovery's Sweet Spot section in Chapter 6.

If you were not just born, or haven't just had a stroke, do you still have access to BDNF? Yes, stroke survivors can produce BDNF well after the subacute phase. In fact, everyone can produce BDNF at any point in their life. But it takes work. The way to pump the brain full of BDNF is with exercise.

Both cardiovascular (heart and lung) and resistance (muscle) training will bathe the brain in BDNF. So, along with all the other benefits to exercising after stroke (see Chapter 5: Elements of Exercise Essential to Recovery), you will also be helping your brain to more easily rewire.

What Precautions Should Be Taken?

The translation of these stroke recovery concepts from animals and humans has only begun. The *"benchside* (in the lab) *to bedside* (with the stroke survivor)" testing is ongoing. Researchers still have work to do, but it is not too soon for clinicians to study this basic animal research and think about how it might influence their clinical decisions.

USING THE WISDOM OF ATHLETES

One group of people knows the secrets of improving physical movement more than any other: *athletes.* The definition of athletes is broadened here to include anyone who uses the full range of physical movement in their career or as their passion. This may include dancers, martial artists, acrobats, yoga instructors, and many others. The secrets of recovery from stroke are hidden within the wisdom of these athletes. This wisdom comes from thousands of years of athletes pushing the boundaries of athletic performance.

Stroke survivors are low-level athletes playing a high-stakes game. Much of what is essential to the improvement of athletic ability is also essential to the process of recovery from stroke.

Here is a list of things athletes and stroke survivors have in common:

- Both want and need to move better. They *do* have that in common!
- Both benefit from cardiovascular (heart/lung) and weight (resistance) training.
  - Survivors need more energy because stroke often causes a lack of coordination. Less coordination means less efficient movement, which means more effort is needed to accomplish tasks.
  - Exercise stores energy. And survivors need energy because rehab is hard, physical work.

— Exercise releases **BDNF** into the brain that promotes brain plasticity. BDNF helps all forms of learning, including relearning how to move after stroke.

- Both use neuroplasticity ("rewiring" of the brain) to move better.

— We don't look at athletes and say, "Look at the size of that guy's motor cortex! That thing is HUGE!" We don't say it because the change is in the brain and we can't see it. The brain is where the exquisite movement of athletes is stored. These areas of the brain that control movement can be made larger, in both survivors and athletes.

- Both learn to move by moving; no one else can learn the movement for them.

- Both benefit from working on the exact skill in which they're interested.

— The brain cares if you care. Do what you love to recover so you can recover what you love to do.

- Both benefit from "a lot" of focused and demanding practice.

— The brain will turn into the tool you need. But to adequately change the brain requires a lot of practice. This work can be **massed practice** (many hours a day in a row), or **distributed practice** (many hours a day, but the hours of practice are broken up, or distributed, over the course of the day). Note that in both massed and distributed practice intermittent rest is required. Rest is essential to the recovery process.

- Both need to measure progress to improve. From tracking their speed to their batting average, athletes constantly measure progress. Athletes are looking for small but important advantages. Survivors also benefit from measuring small changes in ability. Small changes can be important by themselves and/or provide an opportunity to achieve larger changes.

- Both benefit from goal setting.

- Both benefit from **mental practice**.

— Athletes mentally practice (imagine) specific movements in their sport. Survivors can benefit from mental practice, as well. (See the section titled Imagine It! in Chapter 4.)

- Both need coaching. Great coaches help athletes and survivors go way beyond expectations. Great therapists are great coaches.

- Both know that the more they challenge themselves, the more progress they will see.
- Both benefit from an upward spiral of success. Successful completion of one goal leads to new challenges and new successes.
- Both benefit from training on the edge of their current ability.
- Neither athletes nor survivors gain from belief in a **plateau**. What do you call an athlete who believes in a plateau? Retired. Athletes and survivors who accept a plateau create a self-fulfilling prophecy, limiting their potential.

How Is It Done?

Much of what applies to athletic training is useful to the recovery of stroke survivors. Survivors and athletes share the same goal: to get better. The stakes may be higher for stroke survivors but the quest is the same. Learn from athletes; learn from their training techniques and be inspired by their extraordinary level of commitment.

Here are some examples of the elements of athletic training covered in this book:

- **Cardiovascular** exercise (see The Ultimate Stroke Recovery Drug, later in this chapter)
- Weight training (see the section Weight Up! in Chapter 5)
- **Mental practice** (see Imagine It! in Chapter 4)
- Stretching (see the section Don't Shorten in Chapter 3)
- Development of a training plan (see Plan Your Work and Work Your Plan, at the beginning of this chapter)
- Measurement of progress (see Measuring Progress, later in this chapter)
- Not accepting plateau as anything but temporary (see the section Say No to Plateau, earlier in this chapter)
- A healthy diet (see Eat to Recover in Chapter 6) and sleep (see Fight Fatigue in Chapter 8) to improve
- The use of the **neuroplastic** process to turn their brains into movement machines (see Use Your Fantastic Plastic Brain, earlier in this chapter)

It is important to understand the kinship between you and the training athlete. When you need direction, inspiration, or a window on how to train, look to athletes for guidance. Their trial-and-error experimentation over thousands of years provides vital insight. Much of what is known about the development of muscle, **cardiovascular** strength, coordination, balance, and every other aspect of human movement is based in athletic training.

Many of the magazine articles, research articles, and books on athletic achievement and training can be used to direct recovery from stroke. As the quest for recovery from stroke continues, you can use the essential elements of athletic training in your recovery. Also, athletes are role models of dedicated training. If an athlete were to focus on recovery, that athlete would dream about recovery and plan their days around therapy.

What Precautions Should Be Taken?

Athletes are athletes and stroke survivors are not. While the analogy is helpful to educate and motivate, it is not intended to encourage unhealthy risk taking. And that risk may halt progress. If an athlete pushes too hard and is injured they run the risk of slowing their progress toward their goals. If a survivor pushes too hard, the resultant injury could cause two things:

1. Halt recovery

2. Begin a cascade of events that leads to an overall decrease in health. For example, the injury requires rest, which reduces cardiovascular health, decreases muscle strength, and increases weight gain. All of this puts the survivor at risk for other **comorbidities** and could increase the risk of stroke.

As stated before in the chapter, *stroke survivors are low-level athletes playing a high-stakes game.* Injury for survivors comes with higher stakes as well. Consult your doctor and physical or occupational therapist prior to adding any athletic training concepts to your personal training regimen.

THE ULTIMATE STROKE RECOVERY DRUG

Doctors say it all the time: "If exercise were a pill, it would be the most prescribed drug in the world." Being in shape is vital to recovery after stroke.

- *Recovery takes a lot of energy.*
- *Neuroplasticity takes a lot of energy.*
- *Living your life takes a lot of energy.*

Living Life After Stroke Takes a Lot of Energy

Stroke survivors take twice as much energy to live their life than before the stroke. There are many factors that contribute to the increased energy demand. These factors include:

- Moving when movement is uncoordinated (brain problem)
- Moving with a weak side (muscle strength problem)
- Medications prescribed after stroke that can sap energy

Many daily activities, most notably walking, take twice the amount of energy compared to people who've not had a stroke. Not only do survivors typically need twice as much energy to do most activities, they also tend to be much more out of shape after their stroke than before. Survivors have, on average, half the amount of cardiovascular strength as age-matched, healthy people who are out of shape. The same is true with muscle strength. Everything a stroke survivor does takes twice as much energy, but they possess half as much energy. So, survivors must exercise just to maintain enough strength to live their life. Survivors are also battling the natural decline of muscle and cardiovascular strength that comes with aging.

Recovery Takes a Lot of Energy

Research strongly indicates that exercise increases a stroke survivor's chance of becoming more functional. Also, exercise is essential to storing enough energy to continue recovering.

Here are some reasons that that an exercise program should include both cardio and strength-training exercises:

- After stroke, survivors tend to get less of a natural cardio workout in their everyday life. Because walking, bicycling, jogging, and so on, are limited after the stroke, survivors do them less. Try to counteract this reduction in everyday cardio exercise by doing safe and challenging planned cardio exercises. Walking is usually the best choice. But if walking is limited or cannot be done, review other cardio options in the section Hard but Safe in Chapter 6.

- Stroke survivors need more cardiovascular strength than other folks their age, because a stroke causes many activities—especially walking—to require more energy because movement is less efficient.

- There is more chance of a stroke survivor having a second stroke than there is for people having a first stroke. Maintaining strong muscles and healthy heart and blood vessels is vital to reducing the risk of another stroke.

- Strength training, done correctly, can increase mobility (i.e., walking, wheelchair mobility) and make transfers easier (lying to sitting, sitting to standing, etc.).

- Rehabilitation efforts toward stroke recovery require stamina. Short-term bursts, as well as day-long amounts of energy, are required. Motivation means little when you've exhausted your energy and are too tired to try.

- Weight gain increases the risk of diabetes and blood vessel and heart disease. Muscles burn calories, even at rest. This is not true of other forms of tissue. For example, fat burns no energy (calories). Maintaining strong muscles and healthy heart and blood vessels is vital to maintaining optimal weight.

- As crazy as it may sound, exercise increases energy levels.

- Exercise can increase the amount and quality of sleep you get. The better the sleep, the more energy you can put toward recovery.

Neuroplasticity Takes a Lot of Energy

Learning how to move better involves the development of new connections between neurons (nerve cells) in the brain. Every time a neuron communicates with another neuron in the brain, it takes energy. It also takes energy to build the branches of neurons (called dendrites) as well as the connections between neurons (synapses). The amount of energy it takes to drive neuroplasticity is tremendous. Even when learning involves no movement, changing the brain is energy intensive. Consider how exhausting studying can be. And academic study doesn't have the added burden of hard physical movement. The kind of learning that is done to recover movement after stroke is called **motor learning**. It happens in the same area of the brain as learning algebra or chemistry or any other academic subject: the cortex. The cortex is the very thin outer shell of the brain where most learning occurs. Survivors must not only change their cortex, they have to use very difficult movement to drive that change.

How Is It Done?

Have a physical or occupational therapist design a workout that will be challenging and safe. Let the therapist know, up front, that you want an exercise program that can (eventually) be done safely at home. A physical therapist can provide cardio and resistance exercises that will benefit your walking and overall fitness. Ask for an at-home exercise program that

- Is safe
- Has progression built in so that the workout remains challenging over the long haul
- Challenges your muscles and your cardiovascular system

Therapists should be able to develop an at-home program with one to three visits. The therapist calls this sort of at-home therapy a **home exercise program** (HEP; see Get a Home Exercise Program in Chapter 5).

Being in shape is essential to recovery and has been a lifestyle choice for many folks after their stroke. Going to the gym, doing physical work (e.g., gardening, housecleaning), and walking instead of driving are all choices that can get folks into better shape. The more strength that can be stored, the more energy can be directed toward recovery. This extra energy can propel an upward spiral of more energy and more strength, which can lead to more recovery, more effort toward exercise, and so on.

Exercise should not necessarily focus totally on the affected ("bad") side. Stroke survivors can benefit from exercising all four limbs, developing cardiovascular endurance, balance, strength, and agility. Of course, involving the "bad" side is always a good idea. But exercise of the "good" side will help build strength and stamina so that the whole body can recover.

What Precautions Should Be Taken?

There are risk factors with every form of exercise, so consult your doctor prior to changing or starting a new exercise program. Your doctor and a therapist trained in stroke therapy will be able to direct you to the correct mix of exercises. These exercises will be designed to be safe and specifically designed to promote *your* recovery. Make sure that the exercises are stroke specific. Many "exercise professionals" are not qualified to develop an exercise program for the specialized needs of survivors. Stroke survivors need therapists to develop an exercise program that will help with the specific needs required for stroke recovery. And, above all, therapists can design programs that are safe.

MEASURING PROGRESS

How do you know if you are recovering? How do you know if you've achieved one of your goals? Some aspects of recovery from stroke are easy to measure. The first time you walk, climb stairs, or write your name are all milestones that should be celebrated. These examples are easy to observe and identify. "I walked for the first time today!" Everyone understands what happened and is willing to give kudos for the accomplishment. Medical staff, therapists, family members, and friends are there to thrill at the gains made. As recovery continues, attaining goals will generally prove more subtle and harder for most folks to see. Walking a little bit faster may mean you can cross the street safely, but it may not be seen by the world as significant. This is one of the reasons that measuring progress is so important. Accurate measurement of progress will reveal small but important gains. Small incremental steps toward recovery may mean:

- The difference between independence and dependence

- The difference between progress toward recovery and ending progress completely

- The beginning of new skills, which allow for new challenges, which in turn allow for new gains, and so on

You may be progressing greatly, but you don't see it. It is hard to accurately remember where you were a week, a month, or a year ago. There is a tendency to make judgments based on where you were yesterday. Maybe yesterday was a really good day and you made great progress. Maybe today is a really bad day and you actually got a little . . . worse. Many folks will give up after having had a bad day, or a series of bad days: "I'm not getting better, so why should I keep this up?" It may be that you are simply unable to see progress because the day-to-day changes are too small to detect. Relying on memory makes you unable to "see the forest through the trees." Recovery should be judged by what happens over an extended arc of time. It's like the stock market. You would put yourself through a lot of stress (and some people do!) with day-by-day details of how your stocks are doing. Investors in the stock market know that what is important is the overall upward trend. Both stocks and stroke recovery involve collecting short-term information in order to see long-term trends.

Any person trying to learn any new skill has benchmarks that they feel they have to meet or exceed. Athletes use clocked speed, amount of weight lifted, batting average, and other measures to determine progress. Musicians have recitals as well as the ability to play new chords, songs, or pieces. The need to measure progress is just as great for stroke survivors. Here are some facts about measuring the progress of your recovery:

- Effective interventions can help you recover faster than you ever imagined. But determining the effectiveness of an intervention requires accurate measurement.
- If your measurements *do* show progress, you will be more motivated to continue.
- Honestly and accurately gauging *lack* of progress is an essential part of your recovery effort, as well. Interventions that are not effective are a waste of time, money, and effort.
- Measuring progress will reveal gains (or losses) that you might not otherwise see.
- Measuring progress will help you determine if your mix of techniques, exercises, modalities, and so forth, is working.
- In short, measuring progress will determine what is working—and what is not.

If a treatment, modality, exercise, or technique is working, keep it. If something is not working, it should be ruthlessly pitched. The key is accurately measuring the effectiveness of your overall recovery strategy. Because all interventions affect each other, you are not really evaluating individual interventions. Rather, you are measuring your current mix of interventions.

How Is It Done?

Without accurate data, assumptions about recovery are nothing more than guessing. Imagine a researcher scratching his head and saying, "Boy, I dunno. I *think* they're getting better." It would certainly lack merit!

You do not need complicated data collection tools and a lot of computing power to measure progress. There are easy ways of measuring progress that are inexpensive and accurate. No matter what is measured or how it is measured, recording, either through notes (e.g., "I walked three blocks today in five minutes") or by other methods (e.g., viewing a videotape of you walking), will allow you to accurately compare the past to the present. In short, measurement can be done efficiently, simply, and with modest expertise and little equipment.

Here are some ways to measure progress that take little training and equipment:

- *Timing how quickly something can be done:* From walking a specific distance, to saying a sentence, everything can be timed. Timing can be of two speeds; the fastest possible speed and/or "self-selected" speed. Self-selected speed is the speed that is comfortable and natural. Self-selected speeds have the advantage of more accurately assessing speed of an activity in a real-world, normal, and natural way. Timing the fastest possible speed has the advantage of determining the very edge of your ability.

- *Timing how long something can be done:* The length of time that an activity can be performed can reveal valuable information about endurance. For instance, the ability to propel a wheelchair for four consecutive minutes today is better than the two minutes you were able to do last week.

- *Observation as evaluation:* Using a mirror can provide valuable, real-time feedback as to the nature of the quality of movement. This sort of measurement is inherently subjective, but can provide valuable insight into strengths and deficits.

- *Videotaping different tasks:* Video can provide a viewable historical account of progress.

- *Audio- or videotaping speech:* Progress toward improving speech can be evaluated with an audio recording. Videotaping speech has the advantage of seeing the quality of movement of the mouth. Sometimes, however, it is better to not view the speech, but rather evaluate speech only by the quality of the sound. This is because while mouth movements may not be pretty, "ugly" movement may produce the best speech. This is true in expressive aphasia (difficulty speaking) that involves dysarthria. Dysarthria is when the muscles of the mouth don't work well because of damage to the area of the brain that moves the mouth. People with dysarthria may use "ugly" mouth movement in order to produce the most understandable speech.

- *Counting repetitions:* The number of times a particular exercise is performed can indicate muscle strength and endurance.

- *Measuring distance:* Measuring the distance walked is the most obvious example, but there are other aspects of recovery that can be assessed by measuring distance. For instance, the distance reached across a table with the hand, the length of a single step, and measuring the number of inches the fingers can spread apart can all be used to measure progress.

- *"Task-specific" measurement:* You can measure whatever task you are doing, from painting to washing dishes. When attempting to measure how well you are doing in a specific task, ask yourself a simple question: *How would I have measured this on the playground as a ten-year-old?* Children are constantly measuring who is better at what, and if they are better than they were yesterday. How might you measure, say, painting? How long does it take to pick up the brush and load the brush full of paint? How many times can you accurately (as defined by a previously drawn border) "stay inside the lines" while painting a horizontal line? What about washing dishes? How many plates can you get in the washer rack accurately in 30 seconds? How long does it take to wash five dishes? Once you have that number, record it, and then try to beat it. Whatever you measure, make sure . . .

- *It is measurable.*

  — *Measurable:* How high can I reach my hand up while I'm standing?

  — *Not measurable:* Is my handwriting legible? Legibility is often in the eyes of the beholder—you may always be able to read your own writing, while to other people it looks like gibberish. However, even handwriting can be made quantifiable. For instance, using lined paper you can count the number of times you go "out of bounds" (i.e., above or below a set line) within a set amount of time.

- *It is repeatable.*

  — *Repeatable:* How fast can I walk around my quiet neighborhood block?

  — *Not repeatable:* How fast can I walk around a busy city block? There are too many variables from traffic lights to other pedestrians.

- *Take blood pressure and pulse:* Blood pressure and pulse are indicators of cardiovascular health. They are also important indicators of the progress of recovery. Decreases in blood pressure and resting heart rate (pulse) are positive health indicators. For instance, let's say a survivor is trying to build cardiovascular strength and measures their pulse in January as 75 beats per minute. In February she measures 68 beats per minute. This decrease in pulse rate would indicate that her hard work is paying off. Her heart can deliver the volume of blood needed to "feed" the body with less effort (fewer beats per minute).

Measuring pulse and blood pressure is important for two reasons:

1. Pulse and blood pressure can be used to measure progress toward recovery. Generally, a decrease in both are good.

2. Stroke, whether a bleed (**hemorrhagic**) or block (**ischemic**) stroke, is a very significant vascular event. Monitoring changes in pulse and blood pressure can give you and your doctor valuable information about your cardiovascular health.

See the section in Chapter 3 titled Five Tests You Should Do for more information about testing pulse and blood pressure.

When and how often should you measure progress? The more the better is the general rule. The important thing is to be consistent in measuring and recording the information you collect. Once you have collected your information, write it down in a logbook or calendar. For instance, you may write down the time it takes to walk around a quarter-mile track. Every time you make the walk, write down the time. Your measurement will show less and less time to make the quarter-mile walk. This decrease in time may continue for months. At some point, your times will not improve, unless you change the way you train.

Whatever you measure, and however you measure it, make sure the measurements are "apples to apples." Take the example of timing how long it takes you to walk ten yards. You decide that you're going to walk for ten yards twice, and then average the times. A week later you do the same test, twice, and again average the two times. Make sure that for all four measurements you are wearing the same shoes, walking over the same surface, using the same cane, at the same time of day, and so on.

Recovery options that involve a lot of practice per day should be evaluated in the short term (one to three weeks). Change should be measurable in the first couple of weeks. Other activities, like those that involve increasing stamina and muscle strength, take longer to show results.

What Precautions Should Be Taken?

Measurement works to modify behavior because most people try to beat their previous best. Measurement represents you competing against yourself. Any time there is a competition, there is going to be the tendency to reach for the edge of your ability. This striving can be very productive but can put you in danger. An example would be, "I'm going to beat my best time for walking around the block." This aggressive attempt could lead to less safety awareness—which could lead to a fall. Be aware of your own limitations.

2 Recovery Hints and Tricks

CHALLENGE EQUALS RECOVERY

Stroke makes movement difficult. Overcoming the difficulty creates a productive struggle that propels recovery. *Recovery begins at the end of your comfort zone.* If you eliminate the difficulty, you will not progress toward recovery. This is true with any growth in any aspect of your life:

Challenge = growth.

There is a tendency for some stroke survivors to halt their own progress by only working on what they can. For instance, with their doctor's blessing, they may go to the gym and do weight training — an action with positive intentions. Once at the gym, however, they work with the muscles that they can control with ease, while ignoring the muscles that pose more of a challenge. All muscles should be strengthened, including the ones that are cooperating. But emphasis should be placed on muscles that are not easy to flex and on movements that provide the most challenge. Challenge is the essence of recovery.

There is a tendency for clinicians and some survivors to focus on what works. What works after stroke? The "good" side! This approach makes sense if you want to get survivors safe, functional, and out the door. Focus on the "good" side may help you become more functional; a good thing to be sure. But focus on the good side will not help you recover. If you want to recover, the stroke makes obvious what to work on: *deficits*. Stroke survivors will benefit if they concentrate on what they find difficult, not what they find easy. For instance, if you can make a fist but find it hard to open the fisted hand, then work on opening it. The ability to make a fist needs little encouragement.

But the ability to open the hand is just as important. And, since it is more of a challenge, opening the hand requires more attention. You may say, "If I can't open my hand, then what's the use of trying? It won't open!" If a hand is fisted and hard to open, there are suggestions throughout this book that clinical research has shown to increase movement and improve coordination. See the section The Neuroplastic Model of Spasticity Reduction in Chapter 7, which discusses electrical stimulation, mental practice, mirror therapy, bilateral movement, repetitive practice, and so on.

There are options that give you a fighting chance to regain movements that are difficult and challenging. Embrace them. Ironically, overcoming the challenges left in the wake of a stroke is the best way to recover from stroke! If you eliminate the difficulty and only do what you are now able, you would never relearn how to move better. Challenge drives **neuroplasticity**. Neuroplasticity drives recovery.

How Is It Done?

Make an honest and accurate account of your strengths and weaknesses. Recovery from stroke involves making an honest assessment and a constant reassessment of what needs work. List the things that need work, and make that list one of the tools for navigating toward recovery. Focus recovery on movements that you find difficult rather than focusing on what is near perfect. It's a matter of priorities. Activities that are hard provide greater potential for improvement and recovery. Athletes know this. Athletes launch themselves headlong into any challenge that stands between them and winning. Your recovery will accelerate if you honor the challenges that make up the recovery process.

What Precautions Should Be Taken?

Recovery from stroke is hard work. Devoting effort to movements and tasks that are difficult and challenging takes a lot of energy, concentration, and focus. Sometimes the challenge is so difficult that it takes many attempts before the movement or task is accomplished. While this may be safe for some tasks (e.g., attempting to open the hand), it may be dangerous for other tasks (e.g., attempting to walk). Every challenge needs to be undertaken with safety in mind.

Nothing stops recovery like an injury.

USE WHAT YOU HAVE

After stroke, survivors typically move in predictable ways. This predictable movement is called "**synergistic movement**." Synergistic movement does not allow the joints of the limbs on the "bad" side to move independently. For instance, if a stroke survivor tries to bring their hand forward, their elbow comes up and bends, and the shoulder comes away from the body and elevates. All these movements are linked, and the survivor is unable to isolate any individual movement. This is the way stroke survivors naturally move, and there is nothing wrong with it.

If recovery goes well, synergistic movements will become "unlinked" and individual joints will begin to move more normally. Unfortunately, there is a belief on the part of many therapists that synergistic movement is "bad" movement and should never be done. Therapists believe that using this type of movement will somehow be learned so well that it can't be unlearned . . . like a bad habit. The notion that the movement available to stroke survivors is harmful has an ironic (and inaccurate) subtext: "The more you move, the worse you'll get." This thinking is as misguided as believing that, because babies fall a lot as they learn to walk, they will only learn how to fall and never learn to walk! If you have synergistic movement, use it. This will be a common theme in this book: Movement is good, including synergistic. Movement . . .

- Builds strength
- Reduces spasticity
- Is good for joints
- Increases blood flow to the brain, which then makes learning movement easier
- Bathes the brain in a protein (**BDNF**) that helps the brain learn faster

How Is It Done?

Many therapists feel the need to intervene, often with a hands-on approach, to make sure stroke survivors are moving "correctly." But there are several problems with this approach.

1. Recovery should be **patient driven**. This means that you are responsible for your own recovery. And neuroscience agrees: Only the

survivor can drive their own nervous system (brain) toward recovery. No one can do it for them. If a clinician is required to ensure "correct movement," then the recovery process is taken out of the hands of the stroke survivor. There is simply not enough time (or money!) to have clinicians by your side during the entire recovery process. Clinicians *are* absolutely essential at different times during the recovery process. But much of your recovery is going to happen between periods of clinical therapy. After the stroke, therapy is paid for by insurance for a few months. Once therapy ends, it is not the beginning of the end of your recovery, just the end of the beginning. There is still much work to do. And you will have to do that work without the luxury of having anyone there to remind you of the "right way" to move.

2. Relearning to move after stroke is like learning any new skill you've learned in your life. Trial and error is essential to learning how to move correctly. Mistakes allow for corrections and correcting mistakes *is* **motor learning**. Celebrate the movement you have.

3. There is little scientific evidence to support the idea that having clinicians move the survivors promotes recovery.

Many therapists see synergies as unwanted and to be discouraged. Ironically, using synergistic movement is the only way to eliminate synergies! Research has shown that repeated practice, known as repetitive **massed practice**, can overcome synergies. If done in a way that is both repetitive and demanding, practice of movements allows synergistic movements to melt away. In other words: *You need the "bad" movement to get to the good movement*.

Both the arm and the leg have two kinds of synergies: flexor and extensor synergies. It may be that there is logic to synergistic movement after stroke. Have a look at the following images of the flexor and extensor synergies in the arm. What does the movement look like? (Hint: The brain uses about 20 percent of the total calories we consume!)

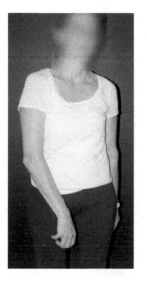 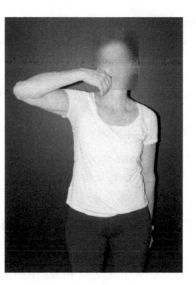

Extensor Synergy   Flexor Synergy

Here are the flexor and extensor synergies for the leg. What does that motion look like? (Hint: You don't need a hint!)

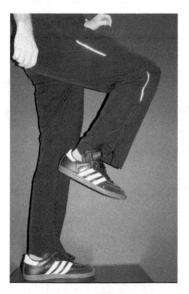 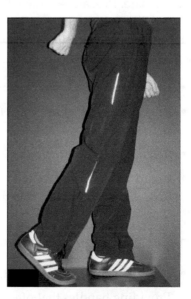

Flexor Synergy   Extensor Synergy

Synergistic movement *is not* bad movement. It is the movement that survivors often have, and they should use it. And what's the alternative? No movement at all. No movement happens in two cases after stroke: (1) The survivor is flaccid (muscles do not work and the limb is limp), and (2) the survivor has spastic paralysis (the limb is frozen with spasticity). In these two scenarios there is typically little recovery because there is no movement to begin the process of gaining more movement.

So, if you have movement, even if it is "ugly" or synergistic—consider yourself lucky! Synergies are a portal to recovery.

What Precautions Should Be Taken?

Use of synergistic movement (the awkward movement after stroke) is not dangerous and will not ingrain those movements. Use the movement you have!

TRAIN WELL ON A TREADMILL

A treadmill is an effective recovery tool for folks who have had a stroke, as long as it is safe. Researchers have found that treadmill training can improve walking quality and increase walking speed. Treadmill training can also boost confidence in everyday walking around the house and around the community by increasing . . .

- Cardiovascular fitness (important in reducing risk of another stroke)
- Muscle strength (important for overall fitness and maintaining optimal weight)
- Balance (important in reducing the risk of falls)
- Coordination (important in reducing the amount of energy it takes to walk, which gives you the ability to walk faster and for longer distances)

Treadmills have the advantage of:

- Providing a safe, straight, flat, and never-ending path on which to walk
- Providing handles that offer endless parallel bars (the bars that stroke survivors hold onto while taking their first steps after stroke)

- Allowing long-distance walking in comfortable indoor settings
- Providing gradation of speed and incline (steepness)
- Allowing for detailed measurement of progress (usually provided as a digital readout about distance and speed on the treadmill's dashboard)

How Is It Done?

First and foremost, consider the safety issues involved in treadmill training given your level of walking ability. Safety issues can be addressed by a physical harpist in one visit. The therapist will review how to safely step on and off a treadmill, as well as evaluate what speed is safe and challenging, given your fitness level. This therapy session should also include information on how to make treadmill training challenging as your walking improves. The physical therapist will review how and when to increase speed, distance, and incline as time goes on.

The next step is buying a treadmill. There are several advantages to having the treadmill in your home:

- The visual reminder of having the piece of equipment in your home
- The convenience: no travel, no traffic, no time lost
- You control the environment, including the music
- You can exercise whenever you are in the mood

A few hundred dollars can provide all the features you'll need. Look for a treadmill that has:

- A motorized walking surface with at least 1.5 horsepower
- The ability to provide an incline (the ability for the walking surface to lift, as if you're walking uphill). Stroke survivors often have "drop foot," which is an inability to lift the foot at the ankle. Increasing the incline of the walking surface increases the challenge to the foot to lift at the ankle. This will develop coordination and strength in the muscles that lift the foot
- Handrails that are comfortable and that you can grasp quickly if needed
- An auto shut-off button that allows you to shut off the treadmill quickly. Look for treadmills that have a tethered cord that you attach

to your clothes, which automatically shuts off the treadmill if you lose your balance

• Easy-to-read digital numbers

Always try out the treadmill before you buy it. Wear the same clothes and shoes you would normally use on the treadmill.

The question of where to place a treadmill requires some thought. There are the considerations of space and where in your home is appropriate to do the hard work of improving your walking. Before you buy a treadmill, measure the length, width, and height of the space where you expect to place it. There is also the question of distractions. If you put a treadmill in an area where there is a TV, radio, or other distractions, is this a good thing or a bad thing? Some therapists believe that stroke survivors should focus only on their walking. Other therapists believe that, since real-world walking involves a variety of distractions (e.g., TV, conversations, phone, traffic noise), the training should involve similar distractions. Alternatively, consider joining a gym (see the section Space to Focus—The Community Gym in Chapter 5) that has treadmills. The money you save on the treadmill purchase can be put toward a gym membership.

If your stroke caused a limp, treadmill walking will not necessarily decrease it if you do not try to look at and attempt to correct the quality of gait. During walking you have limited visual feedback because you see your walking from above, looking down toward your feet. You can better evaluate your walking by having a mirror at the end of a treadmill and walking "toward" the mirror.

What Precautions Should Be Taken?

Treadmills are relatively safe for some stroke survivors, but even for stroke survivors who walk well, treadmills have the potential to injure. The best way to determine the safety of treadmill walking for a particular stroke survivor is to have a quick visit with a physical therapist and let their expertise guide you. Precautions should be taken to ensure the proper use of the machine and that the treadmill is used within appropriate cardiovascular limits. Those who use **assistive devices** such as canes and walkers need to take special care. Treadmills are like moving sidewalks that have an electrical motor, which moves the floor belt in the direction opposite of the direction walked. This mechanism provides inherent risks. For instance, if you stop walking, the treadmill will keep moving backward. This is why it is important for treadmills to have a tethering system, so that if the person walking is carried backward by the machine, the treadmill will stop.

Before you get on any treadmill, make sure you know how to slow it down and speed it up, as well as the location of the emergency off button. Understanding how to safely and appropriately operate the treadmill that you use will allow for a safe, productive, and enjoyable experience.

MIRRORS REFLECT RECOVERY

This section is about using mirrors as an "instant feedback" mechanism to self-correct movement. **Mirror Therapy** (MT), a separate recovery tool, is discussed in Chapter 4.

Rehabilitation from stroke involves relearning movements that, prior to the stroke, were done perfectly. Memory (and observing the "good" side of your body) provides a clear image of what the movement looked and felt like. But many stroke survivors have problems accurately feeling where their limbs are in space (**proprioception**). They may also have decreased sense of touch, pressure, and temperature. The question becomes, how can you relearn how to move when you can't feel how you're moving?

One way to determine if movement is being accomplished correctly is to use a mirror. If you walk toward a mirror, you allow yourself instant feedback about the symmetry (evenness) of the two lower limbs during gait. Walking on a treadmill "toward" a mirror allows you to evaluate your gait for long periods of time. It also allows small, real-time corrections of gait. Mirrors can also provide constant feedback when you're not walking; they can be used to evaluate the coordination, potential strength, and health of the entire affected side, including upper and lower extremities and the trunk.

Some stroke survivors are reluctant to look at the stroke-affected arm and hand. This phenomenon is called **unilateral spatial neglect** (or hemi-inattention). Even after they are reminded to look at the hand, they often will only glance at it as if it holds little interest to them. Another phenomenon caused by stroke is called **apraxia**. People who have apraxia move really well but they have little control over that movement. Mirrors can help survivors with both unilateral neglect and/or apraxia. *Once a mirror is introduced, there is often a fascination by survivors with movement on the "bad" side.* This fascination can provide a renewed focus on their quality of movement.

How Is It Done?

Mirrors let *you* be the therapist and evaluate progress in real time. You may be reluctant to look at yourself in a mirror because you don't like to see your impaired movement. But remember, it's only you that's judging.

Mirrors help survivors compare the "good" and "bad" side. As you look at yourself move, ask:

- Do both arms and hands have the same quality of movement?
- Do both sides accomplish the movement in the same way?
- If they are moving differently, what can be done to make the movements more alike?

Look closely at the quality of movement on the affected arm and hand. Try to have the "bad" side copy how the "good" side moves.

Many survivors find it hard to judge where their limbs are in space if they are not looking directly at the limbs. Again, the feel of where the limb is in space, even with the eyes closed, is called **proprioception**. Proprioception is often lost on the affected side after a stroke. Mirrors can help you tell if proprioception is intact. Try this experiment:

- Face a mirror so you can see your arms and hands.
- Close your eyes.
- Have someone move the "bad" arm and hand into a position and hold you in that position.
- Keeping your eyes closed, move the "good" arm and hand to match the position of the "bad" limb.

Now open your eyes and look at yourself. When the limb is seen in the mirror, does it feel like where it actually is? Are both limbs in the same position? The process of relearning proprioception is done using the same principles of neuroplasticity that are used to relearn movement: a whole lot of practice. Constant visual feedback can help to retrain the brain to remember how movements feel.

Mirrors can also be used to judge symmetry in the arms and legs. This perspective can help you assess the health of the "bad" side. These observations can best be made with clothing that reveals as much skin surface area as possible.

As you look at your reflection, ask yourself:

- Is the "bad" arm or leg the same size as the "good" limb?
- Is the skin the same color?
- Do they have the same amount of hair?
- Do the joints look equal?
- Does one look swollen compared to the other?
- Are the shapes of the muscles the same on both sides?

All of these observations can provide insight into the way your body is recovering. Note: When looking at your "bad" side and you notice that it has . . .

- Change in skin color, including redness or paleness
- Shiny skin
- Swelling
- A change in hair growth
- A change in nail growth

. . . and these are accompanied with pain, you may have **complex regional pain syndrome (CRPS)**. This group of symptoms, also known as *reflex sympathetic dystrophy* (RSD), or *shoulder-hand syndrome* (SHS), can hinder recovery efforts. (See the Glossary for a full explanation of SHS.)

What Precautions Should Be Taken?

Inform your doctor about any changes you observe that seem out of the ordinary. Decreased muscle bulk on the affected side is to be expected. Swelling, loss of hair, or change in skin color, however, may indicate something more serious.

THE MIND, THE BRAIN, AND STICKING TO THE TASK

What is the difference between the mind and the brain?

Mind: You. Your free will. Who you are. Your intentions. Who and what you love, and what you love to do.

Brain: 100 billion neurons inside your skull.

Profoundly, your mind decides what your brain becomes. To recover from stroke, your mind is asking your brain to do a lot. Your mind is asking your brain to rewire massively. But rewiring for recovery is no fun. You're not learning anything new; you're just relearning what you used to do perfectly well. And this is a problem because the *brain* will not rewire unless the *mind* is motivated.

A great neuroscientist, Michael Merzenich, puts it this way: "If it's not important to you, it won't be important for your brain (and no positive change will occur)." Another great neuroscientist, Jeffrey Schwartz, simplifies the idea that the brain changes according to where you put your attention. As Schwartz puts it: "The power is in the focus." Put together, these statements provide profound insight into the brain. You will focus on what is important to you. What you focus on helps determine how your brain is wired. Your brain will work incredibly hard to turn into whatever tool you want. But you have to want it. Focusing on things you really want to do will help you recover. Don't just recover to do things you enjoy; use what you enjoy to recover.

So what's the motivation? What do you care about?

Tennis, calligraphy, painting, writing, gardening . . . anything! By the way, it doesn't have to be something athletic like golf, or artistic like making stained glass windows. The motivations can be much more basic and just as profound. Consider these scenarios:

Scenario I: An occupational therapist walks in to Mr. Smith's room. She says to him, "Good morning, Mr. Smith! Today we're going to work on *toileting*. Would you like to work on *toileting* today? Today's task is *toileting*, yay!" What does Mr. Smith say? "Well, I guess I have to toilet. So . . . okay." Everybody has to toilet, but let's face it, it's not very exciting.

Scenario II: The occupational therapist walks in and says "Aren't you sick and tired of your wife transferring you to the toilet?"

Which perspective provides more motivation? It's not about toileting; it's about *independence*. Beyond what we love to do, what motivates us is everything from fear to friendship, and from money to childcare.

Focusing on what truly motivates is one of the many ways that stroke survivors are like athletes, musicians, and other people who use their bodies in incredible ways. Athletes and musicians tend to excel at what they do because they love what they do. And because they love what they do they're willing to practice—*a lot.* What movements do athletes and musicians practice? They practice the exact movements, or parts of the movements, that they will perform during the game or concert. This is called **task-specific training**. Athletes and musicians are great role models for stroke survivors because they demonstrate the value of dedicated practice.

Imagine two stroke survivors that are exactly the same. They have the same deficits, the same age, everything about them is the same.

Passionate Paul is a drummer. His life as a drummer defines him. It is his work but it is also the fabric of his social life. With every rehabilitation effort he makes, he keeps one thing in mind: Get back to drumming.

Go-Along Gary works hard in rehab. He does everything his therapists ask him to do.

Every bit of rehabilitation research and neuroscience seems to point to the same thing: Passionate Paul will recover more. Of course, Passionate Paul has a much harder road ahead of him. Because he was an excellent drummer, his sights are set very high. For the first few weeks after stroke he can barely hold a drumstick. It requires a leap of faith for him to continue on.

You may wonder why you should try doing things that you know you can't do. Research has shown that task-specific training is the best way to improve upon a given task. Therapists are experts at developing the "baby steps" that you need on the way to your lofty goals. You may not attempt the entire task any time soon. Instead, focus on small parts of the task. The therapist may have Paul just picking up and releasing the drumstick, repetitively. Later she may have him tapping his knee to the beat of music. Both of these—repeatedly grasping a drumstick and knee tapping—are important component parts of drumming. Practice component parts of what you love to do. Once you develop the ability to do the component parts, practice the entire task. This sort of practice is known as **"part-whole practice."** Parts of a task are practiced, individually. Once those parts are mastered, they are put together for a more unified whole.

How Is It Done?

When doing task-specific training, it is essential to try activities that you really care about. The more cherished the task, the more focus will be brought to the training and the more brain rewiring will occur. A task's level of importance can be expressed as this continuum:

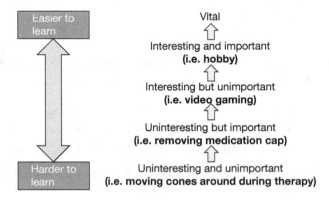

For example, consider George, a stroke survivor who wants to get back to playing golf, which he loves. He knows he'll never play golf again, so he does not think to mention it to his therapist. George is unable to turn his forearm so his palm faces up. His therapist has him hold a small barbell in his hand and let the weight flip until it forces the hand palm up. George could care less and feels like he's spending too much time flipping the barbell. The therapist then has him play a video game where he has to manipulate a joystick by turning his hand palm up and palm down. He finds the game interesting for a while, and then gets bored. The therapist has George pretend to shave with a razor handle with no blade. George finds the task important. He does have to shave, but then again, he could do it with his "good" hand. Then the therapist suggests he start putting a golf ball. At first George refuses. "I'd rather remember my game the way it was." The therapist is surprised to hear that George is a golfer, and encourages him to try. George is told to try to putt one-handed with his affected hand, trying to turn his forearm so he can put the ball straight. George goes home with his forearm aching. "That was fun!" he says. He doesn't even wait for the next therapy session. He goes to a sporting goods shop that evening and buys an electric ball return. *(He starts to imagine returning to golf!)*

What Precautions Should Be Taken?

Task-specific practice is tiring because the motivation to perform the activity is high. Fatigue can lead to accidents. Ask your doctor and/or therapist if the chosen task is safe and appropriate to perform during your recovery.

LET RECOVERY FLOW

Everybody is most motivated by the activities they love. There is a natural tendency to focus on, practice, and pursue activities you love to do. When stroke survivors work on things they are passionate about, it is no longer work, rehabilitation, or exercise. Recovery becomes play. Athletes talk about being "in flow." Being in flow is when you are so immersed in an activity that you lose track of time. When an athlete is in flow, all the problems in life melt away and all that is left is the sport. You can use flow in recovery. Being in the flow of recovery:

- Eliminates self-doubt and self-consciousness

- Allows you to focus on recovery on an instinctive level

- Allows you to focus on nothing but recovery

- Makes recovery enjoyable

- Makes time seem to stand still

- Reduces any aches and pains associated with recovery

- Makes recovery addictive because the feeling of being in flow is addictive

How Is It Done?

One of the most important concepts in stroke recovery is this: **necessity drives recovery**. Define what is essential to your:

- Identity (work, family)

- Passions (hobbies, your art, sports)

- Happiness (playing with grandchildren, attending church)

- Life (cooking, cleaning, grooming)

- Independence (walking)

Walking is a great example of "necessity drives recovery." Everyone knows the importance of walking. Work to recover everything the same way you relearned walking. Identify what is most important to you, and use those things to drive your recovery. If you are working toward goals that you really care about, your effort toward recovery is magnified. Research studies have shown that when stroke survivors focus on *meaningful* activities they get better, faster. "Meaningful" suggests an emotional connection to what is being practiced. If there is no emotional attachment to what you're attempting to recover, you won't see the practice as *meaningful*.

Therapy in a clinic may be effective but not necessarily motivating. Consider playing catch as an example. Therapists often play games of catch with stroke survivors in order to challenge balance, arm movement, and reaction time. This sort of exercise may be fun, and it may indeed help recovery, but playing catch may not hold any importance to the stroke survivor. Therapists use treatments to help make you safer and more functional. But once you return home, motivation may be lost if you are not working on a meaningful goal. The more important the activity is to you, the more motivated you will be. The more motivated you are, the more recovery you'll get. **Necessity drives recovery**. Practicing what you really care about can provide motivation for other tasks that you may find boring. For instance, you may find treadmill walking boring and tedious. But if you are a golfer and treadmill walking follows the yardage of a favorite golf course (a typical golf course involves about five miles of walking!), then you will be more motivated to train on a treadmill.

Sometimes doing the activity is impossible because you just don't have enough strength and coordination, so you take the small steps necessary toward building strength and coordination. Even when you are taking the small steps toward the meaningful activity, the activity should always be in view. This may involve having the tools of that activity visible. Even if you are unable to achieve any part of the activity right now, the meaningful goal should be the guiding light as you move toward that goal.

What Precautions Should Be Taken?

Incorporating activities that you find meaningful into the process of rehabilitation is a positive move, as long as those activities are safe. If you loved to mountain climb prior to the stroke, then pursuit of that particular passion probably won't be safe—in the short run at least! Attempt cherished activities with common sense. The stroke survivor should stay within his or her skill level and make safety the number one priority.

THE RECOVERY CALENDAR

Appointment calendars keep people organized and on schedule. Important appointments, including doctors' appointments, business appointments, and meetings, are all noted. Your recovery efforts deserve a calendar, too. The recovery calendar will help you stay on schedule, and the act of crossing off the items will be partial reward for all the hard work you've done. Keeping a recovery calendar is an easy way to stay motivated and focused. The calendar itself is a reminder to work toward recovery. Also, a calendar helps you evaluate the effectiveness of your recovery effort, the progress you've made, and the goals you wish to achieve. A workout calendar is an essential part of the overall recovery plan.

A calendar dedicated to recovery will:

- Keep track of successes and failures
- Help establish what works and what does not
- Help spot positive and negative trends in the quest toward recovery
- Help separate effective therapies from lemons
- Help measure progress by providing an accessible and detailed account of the arc of recovery. For instance, you may see that the longest walk last month was 20 yards and the longest walk this week was twice that amount.
- Record progress, which is essential to defining and achieving goals
- Help increase adherence to goals
- Add to the sense of accomplishment as goals are met
- Provide an accurate record on which to look back
- Provide valuable information to doctors and therapists as they help you plan your recovery

Calendars allow you to look back and see what you've accomplished. A calendar can also be used to predict new goals. For instance, if in April you walked 100 yards in a single walk, you might be able to project that you can walk 150 yards by June 15th. You can then anticipate and train toward specific projected goals.

WEEK BEGINNING MAY 12 / WEEK ENDING MAY 18	MON 12	TUES 13	WED 14	THURS 15	FRI 16	SAT 17	SUN 18
Walking	Around the block x 3	Off	Around the block x 3	Around the block x 4!!	Off	Twice around the block x 3	Off
Electrical stimulation	Wrist and finger ext. (15 min)	Wrist and finger ext. (15 min)	Wrist, muscles feel stiff (0 min)	Wrist and finger ext. (15 min)	Wrist and finger ext. (15 min)	Wrist and finger ext. (15 min)	Off
Mental practice	Throwing a ball sequence	Throwing a ball sequence	Off	Throwing a ball sequence	Throwing a ball sequence	Off	Off
Rhythmic bilateral arm training	Arm cycle to fav. songs #1, 2, & 3 (~15 min)	Drumming to "Rockin' '78" album (~15 min)	Arm cycle to fav. song #1 & 2 (~10 min)	Arm cycle to fav. song #1, 2, & 3 (~15 min)	Off	Wiping table with towels to 2 songs (~10 min)	Off
Resistance training (legs)	– Squats 3 sets/ 10 reps – Hip abduction 3 lb 3x10	– Hip abduction 3 lb 3x10 – "Footups" 3 lb 3x10	– Knee-ups 2 lb 3x10 – Hip ext w/ band x 5 min	– Hip abduction 3 lb 3x10 – "Footups" 3 lb 3x10	– Knee-ups 2 lb 3x10 – Hip ext w/ band x 5 min	– Squats 3 sets/ 10 reps – Knee-ups 2lb 3x10	Off

(continued)

WEEK BEGINNING MAY 12 / WEEK ENDING MAY 18	MON 12	TUES 13	WED 14	THURS 15	FRI 16	SAT 17	SUN 18
Resistance training (arms)	Band into elbow ext. 3x10	Band press-ups, pulling forearm out 3x10	Band into elbow ext. 3x10	Off	Band press-ups, pulling forearm out 3x10	Band press-ups, pulling forearm out 3x10	Off
Task-specific training	– Putting golf ball 20 min – Throwing a ball 20 min	– Throwing a ball 20 min	– Putting golf ball 20 min	– Throwing a ball 20 min	– Throwing a ball 20 min	Off	Off
Massed practice	– Foot out 20 min – Grasp release 20 min	– Foot out 20 min – Grasp release 20 min	– Foot out 20 min – Grasp release 20 min	Off	– Foot out 20 min – Grasp release 20 min	– Foot out 20 min – Grasp release 20 min	Off
Stretching	Many times throughout day	Many times throughout day	Many times throughout day	Many times throughout day	Many times throughout day	Many times throughout day	Many times throughout day
Pulse, blood pressure	P = 68 BP = 125/83	P = 67 BP = 127/86	P = 62 BP = 121/80	P = 72 BP = 119/84	P = 65 BP = 127/86	P = 67 BP = 122/78	Off

How Is It Done?

Workout calendars are commercially available in bookstores, as downloads from the Internet, or one can be made using personal computer word-processing programs. A recovery calendar only needs three elements:

1. A row for dates

2. A column for the interventions, exercises, or modalities

3. Columns and rows of boxes to input appropriate statistics

An example of a recovery calendar follows. *Do not consider this example as a suggested course of interventions.*

Use a pencil when filling out your calendar. This will give you the ability to correct mistakes and change future goals.

What Precautions Should Be Taken?

There are no specific precautions that should be taken for the actual calendar. Discuss daily recovery activities with your doctor. Please note that the calendar example provided is not a representation of any existing calendar. Do not consider the example as a suggested course of interventions.

ROADMAP TO RECOVERY

Hypocrites (460–370 BC), the "father of medicine," was the first to describe stroke, transient ischemic attacks (TIAs or mini-strokes), and **aphasia**. His word for stroke was *plesso*, which has been variously translated as a stroke of God's hands, to be thunderstruck, and to inflict with calamity. You can imagine how much the ancient Greeks were frightened and confused about stroke. Stroke has no obvious wound, bleeding, or infection, and is often not painful. But despite the lack of outward signs, stroke was often devastating.

As centuries passed, the understanding of stroke and its treatment increased, while understanding of recovery remained limited. It was not until 2,400 years after Hypocrites that someone recognized the predictable pattern of recovery after stroke. Her name was Singe Brunnström. Brunnström, a Swedish Fulbright Scholar and pioneer physical therapist, wrote a seminal stroke treatment book, *Movement Therapy in Hemiplegia* (1970). In her "six stages of recovery" she describes the predictable arc of recovery. This arc goes from total **paralysis** to total recovery. The amazing aspect of this roadmap to recovery is that it holds up against today's scientific measures. For instance, brain scanning technology reveals that *Brunnström's* **stages of recovery** can be used to predict the amount of damage in the brain. Brunnström's professional career ended in the mid-1970s. Brain scanning technology was first seen in hospitals in approximately 1980. (How did she do it?)

Synergy

After stroke, the limbs tend to move in unusual ways. Sometimes the limb cannot make any one movement without making a whole series of unnecessary movements. Typical movement after stroke, where everything in the limb moves at once—even though you don't want it to—is called **synergistic movement** or, simply, **synergy**. Synergies were fully explained in the section Use What You Have, earlier in this chapter.

Briefly, synergistic movement after stroke involves patterns of movements that cannot be isolated. For instance, a survivor cannot *only* bend only her elbow without a whole bunch of other movements appearing. Understanding synergy and synergistic movement will help you understand the wealth of wisdom within Brunnström's stages of recovery.

Synergistic movement is not bad. Synergies are evident in all animals and all humans—even humans who have not had a stroke. Synergies are caused by "motor modules," pathways of neurons controlling several muscles simultaneously. Although mostly tested in gait (walking), it is theorized that synergies help us do many other tasks as well. Synergies are used to bundle movement so we have to think less about our movements. Synergies make movement automatic. The problem after stroke is that some of the more coordinated synergies are destroyed by the brain injury. What are left are more "primitive" synergies. These more basic synergies are expressed in the movement patterns commonly seen after stroke. As recovery from stroke progresses, these less coordinated synergies become less apparent. What emerges is better, more coordinated movement controlled more and more by the brain.

How Is It Done?

Until Brunnström described the arc of recovery, there was no agreed-upon roadmap to recovery. Brunnström's six stages of recovery provide that roadmap.

These six stages also answer many of the questions that you'll have about your recovery, including:

- Where you are in the recovery process
- What new skills appear as progress is made
- What challenges are in the existing stage (spastic, synergistic, limp, etc.)
- What you are striving for, and how you'll recognize it when you achieve it

Researchers use tests based on the six stages as an accurate measurement of progress. You can, too! As you look back at how far you've come, you'll remember the stages you've overcome. As you continue your progress, you will notice that you are moving through the stages, one by one.

In the first stage, the whole hemiparetic ("bad") side of the body is flaccid, and the sixth stage is total recovery. Here are the six stages.

Stage 1

During the first stage, the whole "bad" side is completely limp. The arm, the leg, the torso, the face (including the mouth and tongue) are limp.

Stage 2

Spasticity (muscle tightness) starts to creep into the "bad" side of the body. Spasticity is generally considered a good thing (at this point) because the affected side is no longer limp. Spasticity signals the beginning of messages getting from the nervous system to the limbs. Stage 2 is also when a basic form of synergies appears. There may be some small amount of voluntary movement available, but only within synergy.

Stage 3

During Stage 3, spasticity is at its strongest. Spasticity may become severe during this stage. That is the unfortunate part of Stage 3. The bright side is that you begin to control the synergies. This means that the limbs can be moved voluntarily as long as the movements are within synergies.

Stage 4

During Stage 4, spasticity begins to decline. In this stage, some movements outside of synergy appear. So, two positive things occur during Stage 4: Spasticity and synergistic movements begin to decline.

Stage 5

Synergies continue to decline. Folks in Stage 5 enjoy more voluntary control out of synergy. Spasticity continues to decline as well. Some movements appear normal.

Stage 6

This is the final stage. If this stage is achieved, movements look normal. Spasticity is absent except when fatigued or performing rapid movements. Individual joint movements become possible, and coordination approaches normal.

Here is a visual representation of Brunnström's stages of recovery from stroke:

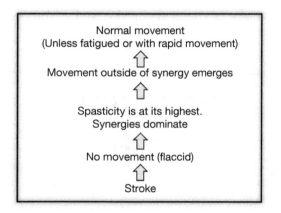

What Precautions Should Be Taken?

Here are some more ideas that relate to the six stages:

- Recovery always moves through the six stages in order. Stages may be brief, but you will go through all of the stages in order. For instance, if you are in Stage 2, you will go through Stage 3 on your way to Stage 4. And you have to go through Stage 4 to get to Stage 5, and so on. A survivor will never go from Stage 5, back to Stage 3.

- Even if you do no work and have no therapy, you still might see progress.

- The process of recovery may be quick or slow and may end. This ending of recovery is what is called a **plateau**. (If stroke survivors work hard, plateaus in recovery tend to be temporary periods. These periods can be used to change what you are doing in order to have progress continue. However, stroke survivors sometimes do not, for a variety of reasons, continue to progress.)
- You will see recovery in the joints close to the body (e.g., the shoulder and hip). Recovery will then spread away from the body (e.g., the fingers and toes).
- No two stroke survivors recover in the same way.
- Recovery of the hand is the hardest to predict. The intricate movement of the fingers and the many different motions of the thumb make any predictions almost impossible. The hand is also usually the last part of the body to regain movement.
- Ability to close the hand will come back before the ability to open the hand.

TIPS FOR THE CAREGIVER

If you've read this far, you know that the message of this book to the stroke survivor is simple: *The highest level of recovery is only possible with relentless hard work.* Caregivers have an equally simple reminder: *Your job is to help that hard work.*

From the shock of first learning that a loved one has had a stroke, and often for decades to come, caring for a stroke survivor can be overwhelming. The sprint of activity in the **acute** stage gives way to the full marathon of recovery. The stroke survivor has to do all of the work of recovering, but the caregiver provides support, resources, energy, and time. All of these elements are essential to the recovery effort.

Stroke is different from other forms of diseases of the nervous system. Most diseases of the nervous system are progressive (i.e., the symptoms get worse over time, such as with Alzheimer's, Parkinson's, and multiple sclerosis). Stroke is not progressive, and stroke survivors have the chance of recovering what the stroke took—with a lot of hard work. The possibility of recovery puts extra stress on caregivers because it is often difficult to know when to push and when to back off. Further stress is added when caregivers believe that the success or failure of the stroke survivor is dependent on their care, encouragement, and support.

How Is It Done?

Next to the stroke survivor, caregivers have the most to gain from the survivor's fullest possible recovery. Aiding in the recovery effort has the caregiver fighting on two fronts:

- Helping the stroke survivor recover
- Maintaining their own sanity

It's a tricky balance and, much like recovery from stroke itself, full of ups and downs. Here are some suggestions for the caregiver

- What caregivers should do for themselves:
  - Contact your rehabilitation doctor (**physiatrist**) and other rehabilitation personnel to educate you in the proper transfer techniques (e.g., from bed to standing or from chair to couch), fall recovery (when and how to help), tricks to facilitate activities of daily living, and so on. A solid foundation in these basics will help the caregiver help the stroke survivor.
  - Keep records of progress made, and note any other pertinent information (lists of medications, important phone numbers, etc.).
  - Keep in mind that many caregivers believe that working with their stroke survivor is an enriching and fulfilling experience.
  - The recovery of a stroke survivor calls for a coach, mentor, teacher, friend, and confidant. Having all these roles assumed by a spouse or any other single individual is a recipe for burnout. Caregivers who wear themselves down are less effective in helping to manage the recovery process. Friends, children, professional caregivers, therapists, and doctors can share in the effort.
- What caregivers should do for the stroke survivor:
  - Provide the infrastructure for the stroke survivor to succeed. This may involve anything from ordering exercise equipment to doing research.

— Allow the stroke survivor to challenge themselves. For example, allow the stroke survivor the time to get the sentence out, rather than finishing the sentence for him, or time to cut his own food, despite the difficulty.

• The caregiver can do three things, every day, that will help keep recovery on track.

— Be a cheerleader. Provide praise. Point out progress. Encourage. Allow mistakes, but also catch the survivor doing things right.

— Be a teacher. Help facilitate proper technique and quality of movement.

— Modify whatever skill is worked on to be challenging. There are many physical challenges that are part of life after stroke. These challenges are, ironically, the best tools for recovery from stroke. Many of these challenges can push the stroke survivor into uncomfortable but productive territory. Resisting the urge to make life easier for a stroke survivor helps lead to gains. There are unmarried stroke survivors who claim that they have recovered because they *had* to recover. There was no one around to "do for them."

After a stroke, survivors are given a tough message. To someone who has not had a stroke, it might sound a bit like this: "You now have to learn to play piano, learn gymnastics, and learn French. And you have to do it all at the same time. Oh yeah, and you've lost your job." Understanding the depth of the challenge of recovery will help the caregiver appreciate the spiritual turning point that recovery becomes.

What Precautions Should Be Taken?

Caregivers who are stressed have a higher rate of depression, illness, and even death than caregivers who effectively deal with the stress and take care of themselves.

An essential resource is provided by the National Institutes of Health (NIH). It is a website that provides a portal to hundreds of pages of caregiver support, suggestions, and organizations. You can find it at www.nlm.nih.gov/medlineplus/caregivers.html

3 Safeguarding the Recovery Investment

REDUCE PAIN TO INCREASE RECOVERY

Long-term pain after stroke is common. Up to 70 percent of stroke survivors experience some sort of pain every day. Pain after stroke can reduce recovery. Survivors with pain have more mental decline, more fatigue, more depression, a lower quality of life, and a general decline in function. There are a variety of treatments for pain after stroke, including medications, things that therapists can do, and things survivors and caregivers can do.

How Is It Done?

The biggest problem with pain after stroke is: *The pain often goes unreported to clinicians.* There is a variety of reasons for this lack of reporting of pain, including:

- **Unilateral neglect**
- **Aphasia**
- An inability to express the pain. For instance, clinicians often use some sort of pain rating scale. You may have seen these as a series of drawings of faces showing various levels of pain. Or perhaps the scale is a 1 to 10 scale. Survivors sometimes have difficulty completing these rating scales.

Stroke survivors should tell physicians and therapists about any and all pain they are experiencing. Caregivers can be helpful in relaying the pain the survivor is experiencing to doctors, nurses, and therapists.

Clinicians sometimes make the mistake of thinking that the pain is related to the stroke because of the musculoskeletal (muscles, bones, and joints) changes caused by the stroke. Of course, musculoskeletal pain after stroke *is* common. But pain after stroke may be caused by something else. So explain it to clinicians in detail so they can make an assessment as to the cause, and treatment, of pain.

The following types of pain are common after stroke:

Shoulder Pain

Here are some interesting "quick hits" about shoulder pain after stroke . . .

- Up to one half of survivors have shoulder pain
- After stroke, shoulder pain shows up within three weeks
- Survivors have a higher chance of having shoulder pain if they also have hemiparesis (arm weakness), sensory problems (proprioception, tactile, temperature sense), and spasticity.
- Shoulder pain is more prevalent in survivors who have *left-sided weakness* than right- sided weakness.

Shoulder pain after stroke can be caused by a number of factors. Included are . . .

- **Subluxation** (dislocation). Find information in the section entitled Shoulder Care 101 later in this chapter
- Impingement (structures in the joint are squeezing or rubbing other structures and cause pain)
- Tears in the muscles and tendons that keep the top of your upper arm bone in the shoulder socket (the rotator cuff)
- Bicipital tendinitis (swelling of the tendon of the biceps muscle near where it meets the shoulder)
- Regional pain syndrome, discussed later in this section.
- Spasticity

Treatments for shoulder pain include . . .

- Percutaneous (through the skin) electrical stimulation: An example of this is Bioness's StimRouter. A fine wire—about the diameter of a hair—is surgically implanted either as an outpatient procedure or in a hospital surgical center (it's minimally invasive and performed under local anesthesia). The survivor uses a hand-held unit to control the amount and type of stimulation to treat their pain.

- Transcutaneous electrical nerve stimulation (TENS): Low-level electrical stimulation done through the skin with electrodes. No muscles contract with TENS.

- Neuromuscular electrical nerve stimulation (NMES): Higher level electrical stimulation where muscles move and joint movement may take place. (See the section Shocking Subluxation in Chapter 4 for information on using TENS and NMES to reduce shoulder pain.)

- Shoulder slings, lap boards, arm troughs, shoulder strapping and shoulder taping: These may help with pain by supporting the shoulder.

- If spasticity is the cause of shoulder pain, the treatments discussed in Chapter 7: Spasticity Control and Elimination will be helpful.

Complex Regional Pain Syndrome (CRPS)

Complex regional pain syndrome (CRPS) is a highly painful condition affecting the limbs. In stroke, CRPS can be caused by the weakness of muscles that no longer support joints the way they should. Typically, this is seen in the shoulder joint due to the subluxation (dislocation) of the shoulder after stroke. Often, this syndrome in stroke is referred to as **shoulder-hand syndrome (SHS).** Although the mechanism (pathophysiology) of CRPS remains poorly understood, the symptoms are clear:

- An arm that is highly sensitive and painful to move and/or touch: Survivors with CRPS that affect the arm often complain that even their clothing hurts where it touches their skin.

- Pain in the leg and foot: CRPS can also affect the leg and foot. The symptoms and treatments for CPRS in the leg are the same as for the arm.

- Signs of CRPS in the arm include any or all of the following:

  — Highly painful

  — Swelling

  — Limb is warm to the touch

  — Changes in skin color

  — Changes in hair growth

  — Muscle weakness

  — Reduced active and passive range of motion

A good way to test if CRPS/SHS is to observe the "good" and "bad" arm side-by-side and note the differences. If any if the above symptoms are evident, bring it to your doctor's attention.

Treatment options for CPRS/SHS include:

- Mirror therapy (see this section in Chapter 4).

- TENS: Low-level electrical stimulation to the affected area. TENS can be used to desensitize the painful area.

- Repetitive transcranial magnetic stimulation (rTMS): This is an emerging treatment for CRPS/SHS. This nonpainful treatment sends pulses of electromagnetism through the skull to the portion of the brain that represents the painful area.

- Imagery/mental practice: See the section Imagine It! in Chapter 4.

- Immobilization: Before anything else is tried, not allowing the limb to move, either voluntarily or with a splint, may help ease the pain.

- Mobilization: Joint mobilization is a gentle passive movement performed to the survivor, with the survivor always able to stop the movement.

- Elevation: Elevating the limb may reduce the swelling and pain.

- Massage: Massage may reduce swelling and decrease pain.

- Gentle range of motion.

- Alternating hot and cold baths.

- Surgery: Discuss this with your doctor.

What Precautions Should Be Taken?

Survivors express pain—40 percent of survivors who initially deny pain express pain once a physical exam is done. Survivors should report pain and clinicians should test for pain. So, the first plan of action for the survivor in pain is not medication or some sort of treatment. It is to *be proactive in reporting the pain* to clinicians. Pain should be reported and tested for no other reason than this: Pain halts recovery.

STAY OFF THE KILLING FLOOR

Falls are a serious health threat to everyone, but falls are especially dangerous to stroke survivors. Here are some scary statistics:

- Up to 70 percent of survivors have a fall in the first six months after their stroke.

- A stroke survivor is up to four times more likely to break a hip than people of the same age who have not had a stroke.

- Stroke survivors are two times as likely to fall, and three times as likely to be injured in a fall, than those who have not had a stroke.

- If anyone over 65 has a fall that results in a hospital stay, they have a 50 percent chance of dying in the next year.

Stroke survivors tend to fall because:

- They have weakness on the affected side of the body. Weakness can cause loss of balance. Stroke survivors tend to lose balance toward the affected side, which can increase the chances of a fall toward the "bad" side.

- They have loss of sensation on the affected side. Loss of sensation in stroke survivors takes any or all of the following forms:

  — Loss of feeling on the skin, like light touch and temperature

  — Numbness in the affected limbs

  — Loss of proprioception, which makes it impossible for the stroke survivor to know what position his leg is in. That is, if a stroke survivor's eyes are closed, he cannot "feel" where the leg is.

Weakness and poor balance control often cause the stroke survivor's weight to be thrown toward that "bad" side during a loss of balance. Once balance is lost, the stroke survivor tends to fall toward the weak side and is unable to brace for the fall with the paretic (weak) arm and hand. During the fall, there is a tendency to land on a particularly vulnerable part of the hip, the part that sticks out on the side of the leg, called the **greater trochanter**. Falling on this part of the leg can lead to a fracture (break) of the upper leg bone or any bony part of the hip joint. Repairing a broken hip is major surgery. To repair a broken hip, either the femur (the bone that forms the top of the leg and forms part of the hip joint) is fastened together with screws and plates, or the entire hip joint is replaced.

These sorts of surgeries are not without complications. You can develop:

- Pressure sores or blisters
- Lung infections
- Urinary infections
- Surgical complications (e.g., tissue infections)
- Orthopedic complications
- Gait deviations (limp)
- **Thromboses** or **embolisms**, which are types of blood clots that can cause another stroke

To top it all off, if you break a hip, you have a greater chance of having another hip fracture.

Hip fracture is only one of the devastating injuries that can be caused by a fall after stroke. Other broken bones in other parts of the body and/or other types of injuries can occur. In many ways falls can be devastating for stroke survivors. Falls can:

- Halt progress toward physical recovery
- Kill (either from the fall itself or from complications arising from the fall)
- Break any number of a wide variety of bones
- Forever end the ability to walk
- Increase the fear of walking
- Reduce the amount and quality of walking

- Lead to wheelchair confinement
- Forever make walking painful
- Lead to a hip replacement or surgery that reattaches the bone

Convalescence from a fall can lead to:

- Clot formation
- Bed sores
- Loss of strength in both muscles and bones, even those not injured in the fall
- Reduced cardiovascular stamina

Physical injury is not the only damaging result of a fall. Once someone has had an incident, the fear of falling again often causes people to restrict cherished activities like shopping, eating out, and attending church. Because of reduced involvement in the community, falls can result in social isolation and depression. Falls also make stroke survivors fearful to work on recovery, especially recovery efforts that involve standing, stair climbing, or walking.

How Is It Done?

Here are some suggestions for reducing falls:

- Exercise regularly. Strong muscles help reduce falls.
- Wear sturdy shoes outside and inside. Do not walk in slippers, flip flops, socks, or barefoot.
- Overall, allow for more lighting in your home.
- Clear away all items that you can trip over. Make sure pets are kept out of the walking area.
- Do not use throw rugs that can slide or move.
- Place often-used items within easy reach to eliminate the need for a step stool.
- Make sure there are handrails on stairs.
- Have your doctor review your medications regarding their potential influence on falling. There is a direct relationship between the number of medications taken (no matter what kind) and the risk of falling.

- There are tests that can be done in the clinic to predict if you are at risk for falls. These tests include:

  — Five-Times-Sit-to-Stand Test

  — Timed Up and Go

  — Functional Reach Test

  — Berg Balance Scale

  — Falls Efficacy Scale

These tests are usually done by physical or occupational therapists. As well:

- Have your vision checked yearly.

- Have a physical or occupational therapist visit your home to make sure your home is as fall proof as possible.

- Consider protective padding. There are discreet hip pads that can be worn inside undergarments to protect hips during a fall. There are many manufacturers producing hip pads of this sort.

- The bathroom is a uniquely hazardous room. Many hard surfaces within a small area combined with wet and slippery floors make bathrooms potentially dangerous. The need to transfer from bath/shower and toilet make bathrooms a challenge to fall proof.

Here are suggestions for keeping your bathroom safe:

- Install grab-bars in the tub and shower.

- Install grab-bars next to the toilet.

- Place nonslip mats in the bathtub and shower.

- Make tiles nonslip with chemical treatments that etch the surface.

- Have adequate lighting on the path to and in the bathroom so that it's easy to see during night-time trips.

- Don't lock the bathroom door in case you need help.

What Precautions Should Be Taken?

The main precaution is *do not ignore this chapter*. This may be the most important chapter in this book. Falls kill. When told of these facts, many people think that clinicians are just trying to scare them. In this case, it is a healthy fear. Take precautions.

REDUCE THE RISK OF ANOTHER STROKE

Many stroke survivors and their caregivers do not know the complete list of possible stroke symptoms. If you've already had a stroke, you have a pretty good chance of having another one. 26 percent of survivors will have another stroke within 5 years of their first stroke. Almost 40 percent of survivors will have another stroke within 10 years of their first stroke. It is essential that you know all the symptoms of stroke, not just the symptoms that were experienced during your previous stroke.

How Is It Done?

Learn the symptoms of stroke. The easiest way is to start at the top of the head and move downward.

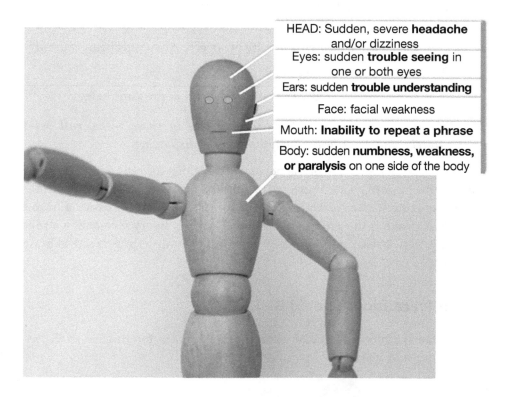

HEAD: Sudden, severe **headache** and/or dizziness

Eyes: sudden **trouble seeing** in one or both eyes

Ears: sudden **trouble understanding**

Face: facial weakness

Mouth: **Inability to repeat a phrase**

Body: sudden **numbness, weakness, or paralysis** on one side of the body

- Skull: Sudden, severe headache and/or dizziness, with no known cause
- Eyes: Sudden trouble seeing in one or both eyes
- Ears: Sudden trouble understanding
- Mouth: Inability to repeat a phrase
- Face: Facial weakness
- Body: Sudden numbness, weakness, or paralysis on one side of the body

There is a quick, easy, and effective way of determining if someone is having a stroke. Developed by researchers at the University of Cincinnati, the *Cincinnati Prehospital Stroke Scale* helps people recognize a stroke by asking the individual to do three things:

1. Ask the individual to smile.
   - Are both sides of the face equal? Is one side of the face drooping?
2. Ask the person to speak a simple sentence clearly, such as: "The sky is blue in Cincinnati."
   - Listen carefully to the quality of speech. Are words being slurred?
3. Ask him or her to raise both arms.
   - Does one arm drift? Are both arms held at the same height?

If the individual has difficulty with any of these tasks, call 9-1-1 immediately, and describe the symptoms to the dispatcher.

React quickly! Some of the newer medications for reducing the impact of a stroke have to be administered within the first 2 or 3 hours after stroke, so recognizing stroke *quickly* is essential to surviving and recovering from a stroke. A stroke is the process of brain cells dying. Every *minute* of a stroke destroys almost two million nerve cells in the brain. Time saved is brain saved.

What Precautions Should Be Taken?

Know the symptoms of stroke. Remember: From the top down—*skull, eyes, ears, face, mouth, and body.*

PROTECT YOUR BONES

Stroke survivors are at a much higher risk for breaking bones than the general population. Stroke survivors have up to four times the risk for breaking bones. There are two main reasons for this:

- People who have had a stroke have a tendency toward high blood levels of an amino acid, homocysteine. Homocysteine can weaken bones.

- The lack of weight-bearing activities such as walking and other load-bearing activities puts less pressure on bones. The decrease in pressure may reduce the thickness of bones, leading to osteoporosis (a process known as **Wolf's law**).

It is essential that you have a plan for maintaining bone health and bone strength. This plan might include any or all of the following:

- Diagnostic tests (bone density tests can be done by your doctor to determine if bones are at risk for fracture)
- Assessment of risk for falls
- Addition of bone-building medications or supplements
- Performance of any of a variety of forms of physical activity, including resistive exercises and a daily routine of walking

How Is It Done?

There are many techniques to increase bone strength and reduce the risk of damage to bones, such as the following:

- As discussed in the section Weight Up! in Chapter 6, resistance training (and or weight training) will build bone thickness (Wolf's law).
- Fall prevention steps will decrease fractures (see the section Stay Off the Killing Floor earlier in this chapter).
- Walking, as part of a daily routine, can reduce bone loss after stroke.
- A variety of medications can decrease or prevent bone loss and have the possibility of increasing bone strength. Ask your doctor about these medications.

- Nutritional steps can be taken to help bone health. These include supplementation with calcium, folic acid, and vitamin B12, plus adequate protein intake. All of these can potentially build bone strength. There is some scientific evidence that vitamins K and D reduce osteoporosis in stroke survivors. Sunlight may help build bones as well.

- There are many techniques that physical therapists can provide, which can improve balance and reduce falls. Have a physical therapist develop a balance training exercise program that you can do safely at home. This should be part of your comprehensive home exercise program (see the section Get a Home Exercise Program in Chapter 5).

What Precautions Should Be Taken?

All of the steps you take to reduce fractures should be discussed with your doctor. Supplementation with vitamins, minerals, amino acids, and so forth may interfere with medications, so talk to your doctor before taking vitamin, minerals, amino acids, or herbal supplements.

DON'T SHORTEN

Some stroke survivors have difficulty straightening their affected elbow because of muscle tightness (spasticity). The elbow is constantly bent, and it continues to stay bent, most hours of the day, every day. After a while, the structures around the elbow joint, including skin, nerves, blood vessels, and other **soft tissue**, shorten. Most importantly, muscles shorten. Once shortened, the tissue will remain shortened forever. Straightening the elbow becomes impossible. The elbow can't even be straightened with the help of the unaffected hand, or with the help of someone else. This inability to straighten a joint is called **contracture**. Contracture eliminates any possibility of the joint recovering its original arc of movement. Once there is contracture, surgery to lengthen the shortened soft tissue is necessary. Another treatment that is sometimes successful is called **serial casting** (explained later in this section). Contracture is a serious condition with serious consequences: If the best possible treatment for you becomes available, contracture will eliminate any possible benefit.

As stroke survivors progress beyond being flaccid (limp), muscles tend to become **spastic** (tight). This tightness can lead to contracture. Safely and effectively stretching the muscles on the "bad" side should be done constantly and faithfully so contracture does not develop. Constant stretching of muscles will help retain the full length of those muscles (and other soft tissue). This will allow you to retain the greatest possible range of motion. Stretching may conserve soft tissue length and protect joint **range of motion**, both of which are essential to any further recovery. Soft tissue length that is maintained will provide the perfect template for recovery techniques as they become available. Other reasons that stretching is so important:

1. **Stretching may provide a short-term reduction in spasticity.** It is common for therapists and other clinicians to believe that stretching reduces spasticity. But because spasticity is a brain problem and not a muscle problem, copious stretching will not reduce spasticity permanently. However, there is some research showing that stretching provides some short-term reduction in spasticity.

2. **Stretching reduces the soreness sometimes associated with recovery efforts.** Much of the recovery from stroke involves repetitive practice, which can work muscles in ways they are not used to. This can lead to something called delayed-onset muscle soreness, or DOMS. This phenomenon usually develops one to several days after the actual practice. Stretching can reduce or eliminate DOMS.

3. **Stretching is good for you.** Stretching is of benefit to muscle and other soft tissue, whether affected by the stroke or not. Retaining flexibility keeps your body young. Stretching will benefit muscles on the unaffected side, the trunk, and in other areas of the body. Bringing a joint through its entire range of motion (which stretching does) also helps to keep the joint itself healthy.

4. **Stretching keeps joints and muscles healthy.** One of the problems after stroke is that the limbs are not moved through their normal **range of motion** (ROM). ROM refers to the complete arc of available, nonpainful movement of a joint. For example, at the elbow, the ROM would be from the elbow fully bent to the elbow fully straight. In folks who have not had a stroke muscles and joints are taken through their full ROM many times a day. Stroke often impedes joints on the "bad" side going to their natural ROM. Muscles and joints are designed to move. Stroke tends to keep muscles and joints static. The more joints and muscles are moved after stroke, the healthier they remain.

5. **Stretching makes every movement easier.** Muscle uses spasticity to protect itself from being torn. Spasticity limits the amount of movement

a muscle can do. The tightness of spasticity stabilizes the extremity. The good news is that muscle is much less likely to get torn since it is stabilized. The bad news is, the limb is hard to move. Both the flexors (muscles that "close" a joint) and extensors (muscles that "open" a joint) may have spasticity after stroke. But the muscles that flex joints tend to be bigger and more powerful than the muscles that extend joints. The upshot of all these muscles firing is what's known as a "hemiparetic posture."

The typical hemiparetic posture in the upper extremity is with the arm across the front of the body with the elbow, wrist, and fingers bent. This posture is simply the flexor muscles "beating" the extensor muscles every time. There is relatively more spastic pull on the muscles that bend joints than straighten joints. This posture is a defense mechanism for the arm and hand. Consider the alternative. If the arm were limp, it would flail by your side in constant danger of tearing muscle, damaging joints, and bumping into nearby objects. Basic protection comes from some of the spastic muscles pulling the arm and hand near the body.

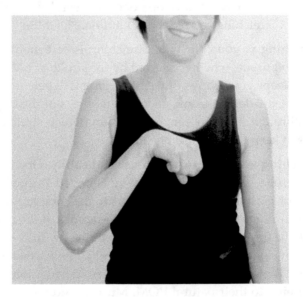

The same is true in the leg and foot. The calf muscles are big and bulky and are actually comprised of two powerful muscles that lift the entire weight of the body while walking. These muscles point the foot downward at the ankle.

The muscle lifting the foot (tibialis anterior) is tiny by comparison. Its only job is to lift the foot at the ankle. This small muscle is in a "spastic war" with the huge calf muscles. If both muscles are in a spastic battle, guess which muscles wins? The "winning" muscles lose by remaining in a shortened position. Over time, the muscles left in a shortened position shorten permanently. This is one of the reasons lifting the foot after stroke is so hard, and why **ankle-foot orthoses (AFO)** are often prescribed.

Note that in both the arm and the leg, there is a "neuroplastic model of spasticity reduction." This radical option that does not require any medications is outlined in the section Neuroplastic Beats Spastic in Chapter 7.

How Is It Done?

To reduce the risk of contractures, perform stretching on yourself, or have a trained caregiver perform these exercises. The joint should be brought through its complete *nonpainful* range of motion several times a day. Generally, stretching is something that stroke survivors can do for themselves.

The best advice available for stretching comes from a plan set up by your occupational and physical therapists. Typically, an occupational therapist would develop a stretching program for the arm and hand, and a physical therapist would do the same for the leg and foot. Ask your therapists for specific stretches that, while remaining safe, are as aggressive as possible and can be done at home. See the precaution section prior to attempting any stretching. Focus stretching on the following muscle groups (it is never a single muscle, but a group that works together, that needs stretching).

Muscles that most need stretching in the arm and hand include:

- The finger flexors (the muscles that make a fist)
- The wrist flexors (the muscles that bend the wrist in toward the arm)
- The elbow flexors (the muscles that bend the elbow)
- The shoulder adductors (the muscles that bring the upper arm close to the body)
- The shoulder internal rotators (the muscles that bring the forearm across the front of the trunk)

Muscles that most need stretching in the leg and foot include:

- The hip adductors (the muscles that bring one leg toward the other at the hip)

- The hip flexors (the muscles that bend the hip toward the chest)

- The knee flexors (the muscles that bend the knee)

- The ankle plantar flexors (the muscles that push the foot down; when standing, this would be a "heel-up" position)

- Toe flexors (the muscles that bend the toes down)

Remember, these are the muscles that need to be stretched, so the stretch would go in the direction opposite of the movement described previously. For example, if you want to stretch the elbow flexors that bend the elbow, then you would stretch by moving the elbow in the opposite direction—that is, straightening the elbow.

A note about stretching the wrist and fingers: If the fingers are stretched without also extending the wrist, some of the muscles will not get stretched. This is because the same muscles that cross the wrist also cross all the joints in the fingers. Effective stretching involves extending the wrist at the same time as the fingers are stretched (prayer position). Conversely, if the wrist is being stretched, then the fingers should be extended.

This is just one of many examples of how stretching may have a bit more complexity than you might imagine. Therapists are experts at taking the guesswork out of stretching. If a high-quality stretching program is developed, it will be effective for the rest of your life. Therapists will be able to develop a stretching program for you in one to three sessions.

Stroke survivors often ask, "How often should I stretch?" Ideally, you would stretch the "bad" side muscles as much as the "good" muscles are naturally stretched. Consider the muscles that bend the elbow. How many times a day is your "good" elbow straightened? This gives us a window on what muscles require to stay healthy. Providing the same amount of stretching as the "good" side may not be feasible due to time constraints. Still, we can assume that an effective self-stretching program needs to be done more often than it usually is.

Another effective treatment to encourage the lengthening of muscles on their way to **contracture** is a long, slow stretch over an extended period of time. The only treatment that holds a stretch long enough in order for muscle to lengthen is called "serial casting." Serial casting . . .

- Involves having the joint casted in a lengthened position, which helps the muscle permanently lengthen.

- Stretches soft tissue by using a series of casts over time. Each of the casts stretches the soft tissue a little more.

- Is usually done by specially trained physical or occupational thera-pists. Serial casting is done in cases where spasticity is very high and regular stretching programs are ineffective.

What Precautions Should Be Taken?

Sometimes spasticity is so strong that muscle turns into a rope-like connective tissue that no longer acts like muscle. This new tissue keeps the joint in a con-stantly flexed position. This is called contracture. If you are unable to take any joint through its range of motion, even with the help of your unaffected side or with the help of a caregiver, consult either a physiatrist or neurologist. There is a window of opportunity when the muscle is spastic (but is still muscle) and when the muscle changes into something else and becomes a contracture. There are a variety of treatments that might decrease the spasticity that is lead-ing you toward contracture. There are two ways to administer medications for spasticity: orally and injected straight into the muscle. Oral spasticity medica-tions often leave patients tired because they are muscle relaxants that affect all the muscles of the body, not just the spastic ones. New developments in the delivery of spasticity medication now allow doctors to target only the muscle groups that are spastic (see the section Give Spasticity the One–Two Punch in Chapter 7). Once contracture has set in, there is still hope—**serial casting,** discussed earlier in this section.

When stretching muscles, carefully follow the instructions of the health-care professional who has taught the stretches. Pain always means, "Stop the stretch!" Even something as simple as **passive range of motion** (having the joint moved without the power of the muscles surrounding the joint), whether done by yourself or by someone else, can be dangerous. Muscles, ligaments, and joints can be torn and veins, arteries, and nerves can be damaged.

There are recent research reviews that question the effectiveness of stretching for the reduction of spasticity. These reviews further question the effects of stretching on muscle length, joint mobility, pain, quality of life, and the treatment and prevention of contractures. But there are still good rea-sons to stretch. For example, the number one cause of post-stroke shoulder pain is not subluxation (shoulder separation due to weakness of the shoulder muscles). The number one cause of post-stroke shoulder pain are adhesions that build up in the shoulder joint (see the next section Shoulder Care 101 for a full explanation of shoulder adhesions). What keeps these adhesions at bay? Stretching. Or at least "ranging." *Ranging* is a term that therapists use to mean taking the joint through its full range of motion. Ranging is done passively, as is stretching. That is, a stroke survivors limb is moved through its available painless range of motion, but some outside force does it. It might be a clinician, a caregiver, or the survivor themselves ranging the joint. Also, stretching provides an immediate—if short-term—reduction in spasticity. This short-term reduction may help your recovery. Stretching feels good, too. The bottom line is, once your therapists and your doctor develop a safe stretching program, the biggest precaution is not stretching enough!

SHOULDER CARE 101

Many stroke survivors have shoulder pain. Even when someone has not had a stroke, the human shoulder joint is vulnerable. This is because the shoulder joint is designed for movement, not strength. After stroke, the muscles that normally keep the shoulder stable are often too weak to hold the joint in place. This can lead to subluxation (dislocation) of the shoulder. Subluxation can lead to painful and limited movement, as well as joint damage.

Because of the weakness of the muscles that surround the shoulder joint, the shoulder should be cared for. This care should begin as soon as the survivor is medically stable and should include passive range of motion (PROM) where the arm is gently and safely moved for the survivor. Also helpful to protect the subluxed shoulder is positioning and supporting the arm both at rest and during any attempted movement. Caregivers and clinicians should take care not to use the affected arm during transfers (e.g., sitting to standing). It is not uncommon for a well-meaning helper to do damage to the vulnerable subluxed shoulder because they use the affected side arm for leverage during transfers.

Even if no dislocation has occurred, the shoulder can be a problem after stroke. Many shoulder problems after stroke are caused by the reduction in overall shoulder movement. In healthy individuals the shoulder is moved in many different ways throughout the day. After stroke the shoulder is often postured in one way for much of the day. The typical way the arm is held after stroke is across, and close to, the chest. The shoulder joint is usually held like this because of:

- Limited strength of the muscles that move the arm away from the body
- Spasticity that makes the joint difficult to move
- Stiffness and pain that limit movement

Often after stroke the shoulder joint is no longer being moved through its normal range of motion.

- **Limited movement in the shoulder joint allows adhesions to build up.** All your joints need to be moved to stay healthy. After stroke, limited movement allows for a build-up of tissue (called adhesions) in the joint. In fact, the main cause of shoulder pain after stroke is adhesions that build up in the joint due to lack of normal movement. Moving the joint through its entire arc of potential movement is important to reduce adhesions. This sort of movement is called "passive ranging." Passive ranging involves the survivor moving the "bad" arm with the "good" arm, or by having someone else move the bad arm for them.

- **Limited movement in the shoulder joint causes tightness in the shoulder joint.** Soft tissue (muscle, nerves, blood vessels, etc.) around the joint shortens over time, which makes movement even more difficult. Because movement is difficult, the shoulder is moved less. Because the shoulder is moved less, the soft tissue becomes even shorter and muscle strength declines.

These factors can make movement uncomfortable, painful, and difficult. In some cases, the soft tissue shortens and adhesions build up so much that movement at the shoulder is impossible. When shoulder movement is limited because of adhesions the shoulder is said to have a contracture. Other terms that are used for this limited shoulder movement are "adhesive capsulitis" and "frozen shoulder." The loss of normal shoulder movement and other negative aspects brought to bear on the shoulder by stroke (e.g., reduced blood flow, muscle atrophy) can magnify shoulder pain after stroke. Also, the shoulder joint can be at risk because people will attempt to help you move by grabbing the "bad" arm, which can injure the shoulder joint.

Probably the worst stressor on the shoulder joint is delivered with pulleys. Pulleys are handles attached to ropes. The ropes are attached to a wheel so that if you pull downward on one handle, the other handle (with the other arm and hand holding it) goes upward. Pulleys are available in most rehabilitation gyms. Therapists often use them to help patients with different disorders (not just stroke) "range" themselves (self-stretch). Pulleys can be dangerous for the weak-side shoulder of stroke survivors. Unless a doctor specifically suggests pulleys, decline their use. Other forms of aggressive "ranging" (putting the joint through, and beyond, its range of motion) with the aid of your "good" side, or with the aid of another person or machine, should be considered cautiously. Aggressive ranging of the shoulder joint can damage the joint. Keep in mind, however, that proper, nonpainful stretching of the shoulder joint is necessary after stroke. The shoulder should be part of a comprehensive stretching program. Your stretching program should take all the joints on the affected side through their full, safe, and nonpainful passive range of motion.

How Is It Done?

It is important to focus attention on the affected shoulder to prevent injury, increase coordination, and keep muscles strong. This attention will allow for the largest possible potential recovery of shoulder movement. Here are strategies that can help to protect the shoulder:

- Kenisiotaping (also known as physiotaping or simply taping or strapping): This may protect the shoulder and allow for correct movement. Note that there is very little research indicating that shoulder taping after stroke helps shoulder movement or shoulder function. However, while it's worn, tape may help reduce pain. Many therapists view taping as a promising treatment option for shoulder pain after stroke.

- Positioning techniques: Positioning the shoulder when the arm is at rest in order to protect the joint.

- Shoulder slings: There is limited evidence that shoulder slings can help shoulder function and protect the shoulder.

- Strengthening surrounding muscles: The best way to protect the shoulder joint is to strengthen the muscles around it and adequately and gently stretch the joint. Occupational and physical therapists are experts in exercises that aid the shoulder joint. Exercises that build muscle to support the shoulder are essential. Rehabilitation specialists can provide exercises appropriate for stroke survivors. Consult your doctor and rehabilitation healthcare worker and ask them to provide an exercise plan that will help shoulder recovery.

- Many researchers believe that the best thing you can do for your shoulder is increase movement in the hand. The shoulder is, after all, there to get the hand where it needs to go. The shoulder will develop strength and coordination naturally if it is moving the hand in real-world ways. The work of getting the hand functional can have a significant effect on the muscles that control the shoulder. Some therapists and researchers believe that a useable hand will actually resolve subluxation (dislocation) of the shoulder. As the hand is used more, the shoulder muscles are used more. As the shoulder muscles are used, they strengthen, which pulls the shoulder joint together. Ideas to get the hand "back in the game" are discussed in the section in Chapter 4 titled Get Your Hand Back.

What Precautions Should Be Taken?

Consult your doctor regarding any pain that affects function of the shoulder. Don't make the mistake of not consulting a doctor for pain that limits movement. Reduced movement can lead to a downward spiral, causing shortening of the soft tissue that surrounds the joint, which leads to less movement and, in turn, can lead to more shortening of soft tissue. Limited movement can also increase the incidence of adhesions in the shoulder joint. Periodically consult your occupational or physical therapist for proper exercises and other treatments and modalities to help support the weak-side shoulder.

FIVE TESTS YOU SHOULD DO

You will often hear about how important cardiovascular health is. For stroke survivors, the impact of damaged and clogged arteries has already been felt. You might think that having a stroke is an isolated incident. But the truth is that stroke survivors have their stroke to thank for alerting them that all is not well with their blood vessels. Vascular disease is not isolated; it is a disease that usually shows up in the walls of many arteries at once. Arteries are the blood vessels (*plumbing*, if you will) that take blood from your heart and delivers it to every one of the trillions of cells in your body. There are an estimated 30 thousand miles of arterial blood vessels in the human body. Arterial disease can happen in any number of vessels. The fact that some arteries are diseased may not make much difference in your life. But in some organs, like the heart and brain, this disease process can kill you. Stroke survivors know what can happen in the brain when an artery clogs or bursts: stroke. Most people know the impact of this disease in the heart, too: a heart attack. Arterial disease is 80 percent preventable. Here are a few basic steps that you can take to keep your arteries healthy:

- Stop smoking
- Control your diet/weight, blood pressure, and cholesterol
- Control diabetes
- Exercise

All of these will benefit the health of your arteries. Once you put these efforts into practice, follow up by doing some simple tests. These tests will help you determine if your efforts are successful.

One other thing you can do to help keep your arteries healthy: control stress. Stress can cause a stroke. Actress Debbie Reynolds recently died just one day after the death of her daughter, actress Carrie Fisher. The press says she died of a "broken heart" and that is probably true. There is now science that shows that stress can cause stroke and other cardiovascular diseases. But the connection between stroke and stress is indirect. Here's the story: The amygdalae (plural; there are two of them. Singular is amygdala) are small, marble-sized structures in the brain responsible for emotions. In folks who have cardiovascular disease (like stroke) there is more activity in the amygdalae. This increased activity causes more C-reactive protein, a ring-shaped protein found in blood. C-reactive protein clots blood. Blood clot in the brain = stroke. Bottom line: Stress = Increased blood clotting = Stroke.

How Is It Done?

A series of tests that can reveal arterial health follows. Two of them, pulse and blood pressure (BP), should be done during the entire recovery process. They should also be done during each recovery workout or session. Pulse and BP will provide essential information that will keep you safe as you continue to recover. Pulse and BP can also provide information about overall, long-term cardiovascular health and strength. Generally, the lower the numbers for both pulse and BP, the better. Your doctor can provide specific guidelines. Pulse and blood pressure should also be taken during periods of activity and rest. Resting pulse and resting BP are key indicators of cardiovascular health (again, generally, the lower the better). Keep an ongoing record of these two measures. Your self-testing results will provide valuable information for your doctor and therapists, so bring the results with you when visiting health professionals. Knowing, by *heart*, your average pulse and BP will help you know if you are remaining safe.

Here are a few basic tests that stroke survivors can do to keep track of the health of their arteries:

- *Take your blood pressure.* Digital blood pressure machines are inexpensive and easy to use. Bring your machine into your doctor's office to judge the machine's accuracy. Compare the doctor's reading against what your machine says. Your doctor will tell you what normal blood pressure is for you; normal varies from person to person depending on a number of factors, including the effects of certain medications.

- *Take your pulse.* (Many digital blood pressure monitors take pulse as well.) Here is how to take pulse: Look at a clock with a second hand. Place the tips of your "good-side" index and long fingers on the palm side of your other wrist, below the base of the thumb. Press lightly with your fingers, feeling the pulsing with your fingertips. Count the number of beats for 15 seconds. Multiply the number of beats by four. The number you come up with is your pulse per minute.

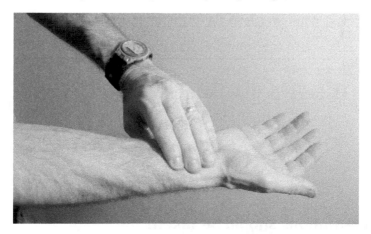

- Ask your doctor what a "good" pulse rate should be under two conditions:
    - *The highest pulse you can safely maintain during exercise.* Much of what is suggested in this book is aerobic exercise (exercise involving the heart and lungs) and aerobic exercise increases heart (pulse) rate. Knowing the safe range of pulse rate will not only keep you safe, but can be used as a training tool. The key to maintaining

an optimal pulse rate during exercise is challenging but safe. You want to challenge the heart (so it will get stronger) but keep your pulse rate in a safe range.

— *Your average pulse when you are resting*. Resting pulse rate is best done before you get out of bed in the morning. Resting heart rate is an important indicator of overall cardiovascular (heart and lung) health.

- *Have your cholesterol checked by a doctor*. It is a blood test. There are at-home blood tests, but their accuracy may be questionable.

- *Monitor blood sugar*. You can do this even if you are not diabetic but suspect something may be wrong with your blood sugar. There are inexpensive, over-the-counter blood sugar tests at your drug store.

- *Take your **waist-to-hip ratio***. Waist-to-hip ratio is the best predictor of cardiovascular death. **Central obesity** (carrying fat around the middle, or an apple-shape, where the waist is larger than the hips) increases the risk of stroke, heart disease, high blood pressure, and diabetes. Carrying fat in the hips and thighs, or having a pear shape, is not as harmful to your health. You can calculate your waist-to-hip ratio by dividing your waist measurement by your hip measurement.

  — Waist: Relaxed, measured around at belly button.

  — Hips: Measure around the widest part of the hip-bones.

  — For instance:

  — Measurement at the waist = 34

  — Measurement at the hips = 37

  — $34 \div 37 = 0.92$

  — Ratios above 0.80 for women and 0.95 for men increases the risk of stroke, heart disease, high blood pressure, and diabetes.

What Precautions Should Be Taken?

Home tests are great. They are convenient, and they tell you what you need to know. But these tests are done most accurately when skilled healthcare professionals do them. Lack of accuracy of machines, as well as poor collection techniques, can provide false readings. If you suspect that a reading (pulse rate, blood pressure, etc.) is cause for concern, contact your doctor or call emergency services (911).

4 Cool Treatment Options

CONSTRAINT-INDUCED THERAPY FOR THE ARM AND HAND

The basis of most recovery from stroke is **neuroplasticity** (see the section Use Your Fantastic Plastic Brain in Chapter 1). There are several ways of activating the neuroplastic process. The most famous is **constraint-induced therapy (CIT)**. CIT is the most researched and the most clinically proven stroke recovery option. In traditional CIT, the "good" hand and arm are immobilized with either a sling and/or mitt while the "bad" hand and arm do a lot of **repetitive practice**. In the clinic, the exercises are repeated for six to eight hours a day, for two to three weeks. Added to that practice is another element of CIT. When they are at home during those two to three weeks, there is added work: Patients have to wear a sling and/or mitt 90 percent of their waking hours. If this schedule seems tough, consider the fact that athletes and musicians often spend multiple hours a day skill building. And they do it year in and year out. A stroke survivor who is trying to recover is just like an athlete or musician; they are always trying to rewire theirs brain by practicing with their limbs.

How Is It Done?

There are facilities that provide structured CIT programs. The most famous is the Taub Therapy Clinic, located in Birmingham, Alabama. This clinic is run by Edward Taub, PhD, originator of CIT.

- Taub Therapy Clinic, Birmingham, Alabama
- Website: www.taubtherapy.com
- Phone: 866-554-TAUB

This clinical intervention is intense; it lasts for either two or three weeks, and it is done multiple hours a day. This therapy is expensive because it requires many hours of occupational and physical therapy, and a therapist's time is expensive.

Another form of CIT is called *modified* constraint-induced therapy (mCIT). Developed by stroke-recovery researcher Dr. Stephen J. Page, mCIT is now available in many facilities across the United States. mCIT is different from traditional CIT in terms of the number of hours a day that are needed to see the treating therapist. With classic mCIT, the stroke survivor sees the therapist three times a week, but wears a constraint on the affected arm and hand for up to five hours a day during active hours when they are at home. Compared to traditional CIT, mCIT uses less clinical hours, with more of the work being done at home. Less time in the clinic makes mCIT a less expensive option. The multiple hours required by traditional CIT makes it impossible for many therapists to schedule. Because the amount of time spent in the clinic is radically reduced, therapists can fit mCIT into their normal working day.

Note that any form of constraint-induced therapy is some combination of repetitive practice (done in the clinic) and forced use (done at home).

The question of how much time is spent on each is flexible and is determined by the needs and wishes of the clinicians (doctors, therapists, etc.) and survivors. This combination of factors helps determine the "dose" of CIT.

Analysis of research has led to an accepted total amount of hours spent of CIT per day as somewhere between one-half and three hours.

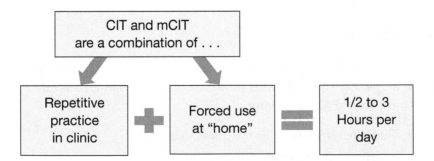

Therapists have been modifying mCIT ever since the mid-2000s to fit their set of skills and incorporate the resources of their particular hospital or rehab facility.

Here is a partial list of facilities that provide some form of CIT or mCIT:

- Kessler Institute for Rehabilitation, West Orange, New Jersey
  Website: kessler-rehab.com
  Phone: 973-731-3600

- Garden State Physical Therapy P.C., Hasbrouck Heights, New Jersey
  Website: marketingconsultant.powweb.com/id11.html
  Phone: 201-998-6300

- Burke Rehabilitation Hospital, White Plains, New York
  Website: burke.org
  Phone: 914-597-2500

- Sunnyview Rehabilitation Hospital, Schenectady, New York
  Website: sunnyview.org
  Phone: 518.382.4500

- Magee Riverfront, Philadelphia, Pennsylvania
  Website: mageerehab.org/rehab-services/outpatient-and-specialties/
  constraint-induced-movement-therapy
  Phone: 215-218-3900

- Braintree Rehabilitation Hospital, Braintree, Massachusetts
  Website: healthsouthbraintree.com/en/our-approach/
  conditions-we-treat/stroke
  Phone: 781-348-2500

- Spaulding Rehabilitation Hospital, Boston, Massachusetts
  Website: spauldingnetwork.org
  Phone: 617-573-7000

- Fairlawn Rehabilitation Hospital, Worcester, Massachusetts
  Website: fairlawnrehab.org
  Phone: 508-471-9322

- CarePartners Health Services, Asheville, North Carolina
  Website: www.carepartners.org/services_atoz_ci.html
  Phone: 828277-4800

- Emory Healthcare's HealthConnections, Atlanta, Georgia
  Website: emoryhealthcare.org
  Phone: 404-778-7777

- Siskin Hospital for Physical Rehabilitation, Chattanooga, Tennessee
  Website: siskinrehab.org/patient/costraint.asp
  Phone: 423-634-1200

- Shirley Ryan Ability Lab Chicago
  Website: sralab.org/conditions/stroke-recovery
  Phone: 800-354-7342

- University of Michigan Health System, MedRehab, Ann Arbor, Michigan
  Website: med.umich.edu
  Phone: 734-998-7911

- Advanced Recovery Rehab Center, Sherman Oaks, California
  Website: advancedrecovery.org
  Phone: 818-386-1231

- Mercy General Hospital, Sacramento, California
  Website: mercygeneral.org
  Phone: 916-453-4621

- Precision Rehabilitation, Long Beach, California
  Website: precisionrehabilitation.com
  Phone: 562-988-3570

- Providence Health & Services Alaska, Anchorage, Alaska
  Website: alaska.providence.org/locations/pamc/services/rehabilitation
  Phone: 907-212-6300

- Manchester Neuro Physio, Manchester, Liverpool and Cheshire, UK
  Website: www.manchesterneurophysio.co.uk/index.php
  Phone: 0161.883.0066

Constraint-induced therapy (and mCIT) will not work if there is no jumping-off point. Research shows that you need some movement in the hand to start with. Here are some of the tests that researchers and clinicians have used to determine if CIT or mCIT is appropriate for someone:

- The ability to actively lift hand, thumb, and at least two fingers from a relaxed (drooped) position

- The ability to release a grasped tennis ball

- The ability to pick up and release a cloth off a table top using any type of grasp/release

There is research that has shown success with survivors with even less movement. One such standard is simply the ability to wipe a towel across a table. Therapists have used similar standards in the clinic.

Can someone do CIT alone at home? Certainly; there are elements of CIT that you can do at home, safely, and with little training and setup. But there are also mistakes that can be made when attempting CIT. Mistakes can make the therapy ineffective and, worse, can put the stroke survivor at risk of injury. CIT should be done, at least to begin with, while working with an occupational or physical therapist. CIT is simply a way to stop, and reverse, what researchers call **learned nonuse**. Learned nonuse is when stroke survivors essentially teach themselves *not* to use their "bad" limbs.

Here is an example of learned nonuse:

You try to open your hand to pick up a glass. But opening your hand is difficult, time-consuming, and clumsy. Every time you pick up a glass with liquid you run the risk of spilling it all over yourself. So you don't try to pick up a glass (all you'll do is spill!). The less you attempt any movement, the

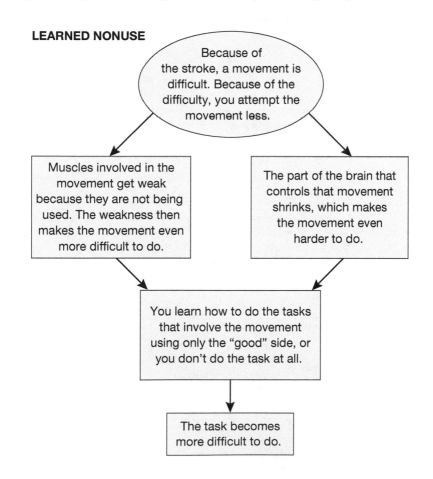

LEARNED NONUSE

Because of the stroke, a movement is difficult. Because of the difficulty, you attempt the movement less.

Muscles involved in the movement get weak because they are not being used. The weakness then makes the movement even more difficult to do.

The part of the brain that controls that movement shrinks, which makes the movement even harder to do.

You learn how to do the tasks that involve the movement using only the "good" side, or you don't do the task at all.

The task becomes more difficult to do.

more the part of the brain that controls that movement shrinks. That's the way the brain works; it is very "use it or lose it." In this case, it's move it or lose it. The overall effect of not using the movement is the movement becomes more difficult. Meanwhile, every time you use the "good" side, everything works great. In a sense you are rewarded for using your "good" side and punished for using your "bad" side. As a result, you use the "bad" limb even less, which means even less dedicated brain power, and so the downward spiral continues. In this way the stroke survivor "learns" not to use the affected "bad" limb. And the brain adds to the problem. After a stroke, the damaged side of the brain gets less active, while the undamaged side becomes more active. Your brain is working against you! But remember, you are in control. Your brain (the object) takes directions from your mind (your free will).

REVERSING LEARNED NONUSE

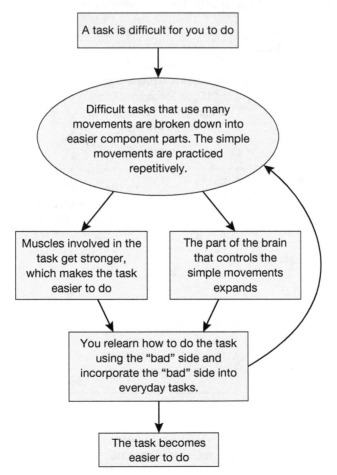

CIT is considered a behavioral therapy. The idea behind behavioral therapies is simple: The way you live your life (behave) changes the way your brain is wired. This is true with regard to any kind of behavior, and is certainly true with stroke recovery. With CIT, the behavior you are changing is "nonuse" of your "bad" arm and hand. More directly, you are behaving in a way that uses the "bad" arm and hand more.

To review: The more brainpower devoted to that movement, the easier the movement becomes. The opposite is also true: As you use the limb less, less brainpower is directed to that movement. The less brainpower dedicated to the movement, the worse the limb moves. Constraint-induced therapy (CIT) attempts to reverse the downward spiral of learned nonuse by forcing you to use the "bad" limb. CIT uses **repetitive practice** of the "bad" limb to promote recovery.

What is practiced are "valued tasks," which are tasks that the survivor is very motivated to do. (See the section titled The Mind, the Brain, and Sticking to the Task in Chapter 2 for more about why valued tasks are essential to recovery.) Small parts of the task, called "**component parts,**" are practiced over and over. As each of the component parts of the task are learned, all the parts are put together and the entire task is practiced. The process of developing component parts needed for one task helps with other tasks, as well. Consider that component part of lifting your arm at the shoulder as part of reaching for a cup. Once the ability to lift the arm is learned, it can be used to do many other tasks, from writing (to get the arm to the table) to turning on a light switch. This process of building small parts of a movement into an effective whole movement is the basis of CIT.

CIT should be taught by a trained rehabilitation professional. Once you understand the basic ideas behind using CIT to recover movement, you can easily use the spirit of CIT and mCIT in other areas of your recovery.

Leg Constraint-Induced Therapy (Leg CIT)

The spirit of CIT is that the "good" limb essentially *does nothing*, while the "bad" limb does all the work. Research into leg CIT lags far behind arm/hand CIT because it is difficult to respect the spirit of CIT *and* keep you safe. Remember, CIT involves constraining, with a sling and/or mitt, the "good" arm and hand. A quick look at leg CIT reveals the problem. How do you safely constrain a leg? How do you have only one limb do all the work and still engage in the primary function of the legs—walking? Leg CIT has another problem.

The core of CIT involves practice with the "bad" side for a half-hour to three hours a day. You can survive this tough schedule when doing arm/hand CIT because you are sitting most of the time. But for much of leg CIT, the survivor is standing. Because it is done while standing, leg CIT provides a significant challenge to endurance. Also, the muscles of the arm are small, relative to the leg. Since the leg muscles are much bigger than the arm muscles, you burn much more energy. This makes the harsh scheduling of CIT difficult to maintain.

Because of these inherent problems, leg CIT is done less often clinically. Clinics that attempt this treatment use similar techniques to those used in arm/ hand CIT. Leg CIT involves a lot of intense exercises for the "bad" leg. The goals of these exercises are twofold. First, the idea is to strengthen the muscles of the "bad" leg so that the limb is at least as strong as the "good" leg. Second, this strategy provides many repetitions of component parts of walking (i.e., **dorsiflexion**, or lifting the foot) to cause the necessary **neuroplastic** change.

What Precautions Should Be Taken?

Make sure, before any CIT or mCIT program is started, that the version that the facility or therapist is using is shown to be effective in research that is published in **peer-reviewed** literature. Facilities and individual clinicians often claim they do CIT. But a closer look reveals that they have watered down the therapy so much that it is ineffective. CIT involves a strict schedule in the clinic and/or at home. CIT also involves significant paperwork. If either of these (often hours a day and paperwork) are not part of the CIT treatment, be skeptical.

DO NOT constrain the unaffected hand and arm unless under the supervision of a physician or therapist. There are safety issues that must be considered when restricting the "good" extremity. Constraining the "good" arm and hand can lead to falls, burns, and other dangers. Note that there is a general consensus that the least amount of constraint possible should be used. In other words: Whatever is used as constraint (sling, mitt, glove, etc.) should be no more than a reminder to use the affected limb. There are inherent risks in wearing, for instance, a sling on the "good" side. If a survivor is in the process of falling and tries to stabilize themselves with their "good" arm, the sling will restrict their movement and the survivor could fall. So the constraint should be little more than a reminder to use the "bad" limb as much as possible. There is a general shift away from a sling and toward a glove or a mitt. A glove or mitt allows for protective extension (stabilizing against a fall) but still provides a hedge against learned nonuse.

Lower-extremity CIT exists but has to be done under the direct supervision of a therapist. Some of the facilities that offer CIT for the arm and hand also have CIT programs for the leg. Never attempt lower-extremity CIT without therapist supervision. DO NOT tie up the leg and/or foot. Constraint of the lower extremity is not done in any form of lower-extremity CIT.

GET YOUR HAND BACK

Generally speaking, the shoulder, elbow, and wrist are simply delivery systems for the hand. That is, the entire arm exists to bring the hand to where it needs to be. If the hand can be used in some sort of real-world way, all the muscles of the arm will work very hard to get the hand where it needs to be. In other words, a useable hand will help the entire arm recover.

But what if your hand does not yet work? Typically, the hand is the last body part to recover. Arm recovery tends to begin in muscles and joints close to the body and move down the limb, toward the hand. Stroke survivors typically regain movement in this order:

1. The muscles that move the shoulder blade
2. The muscles that move the shoulder joint (which moves the upper arm)
3. The muscles that move the elbow
4. The muscles that rotate the forearm (palm up and palm down)
5. The muscles that move the wrist
6. The muscles that move the hand and fingers

Remember, the arm has a strong chance of recovering if the hand is working. But, because the hand comes back last, it is impossible to use the hand to help recovery in the rest of the arm. Recently however, researchers, entrepreneurs, and bioengineers have begun to solve the riddle of the hand. What has come of this research and experimentation has been the clinical use of a variety of gizmos, orthotics, machines, and techniques to "jump start" the hand.

How Is It Done?

How to jump start the hand depends on how much movement the hand has to begin with. Stroke survivors often grossly underestimate the movement in their hands. They tend to think that, since the hand is not useful in any real-world way, any movement it has is not important. But a small amount of movement is important to one thing: *recovery*.

If you have any movement, in any joint, you can build on that movement by using **repetitive practice**. Repetitive practice means using the little movement you have, over and over, to try to "hit the end ranges" of that movement. In the fingers, this would mean opening and closing the fist as much as possible. "Hitting the end ranges" would involve extra focus on the tail end of both of those movements. So you would open the fingers as much as possible and then try to open them just a little bit farther. Then you would try to close the hand and then close it a little bit more.

The movement to open the hand may not amount to much more than the ability to relax the fingers enough to allow the fingers to "relax open." This ability to relax the fingers so they open slightly is important because it takes two to tango. The muscle that opens the fingers has to fire, but equally important, the muscles that close the fingers have to relax. It is this dance between the muscles groups that presents the challenge when you try to open and then close your hand. Once you can open and close even one finger, repeat it for as long as you can tolerate it. Do it while you watch TV, talk on the phone, wherever and whenever. With luck, the other fingers and, eventually, the thumb, will follow if you try to repeat, over and over, the grasp/release movement of opening and closing the fingers.

But what if you have *no* movement? Or what if, as is the case with most stroke survivors, you can make a tight fist, but releasing that fist is impossible? This is where the machines and gizmos can help.

- *Cyclic electrical stimulation:* One sort of machine that you can try uses cyclic electrical stimulation. This is electrical stimulation to, in this case, activate the muscles that open the hand. These muscles are located on the back of the forearm. The machine simply stimulates the hand to open, and then the machine stops the stimulation. On and off it goes usually for five seconds or so of hand opening, followed by ten seconds or so of no stimulation. These machines are relatively inexpensive, and once a doctor or therapist trains you on the machine, you can do it at home. If help is also needed to close the hand, then the machine can be programmed to first open, provide no stimulation, and close the hand. For more information about this treatment see Electrical Stimulation for Frugal Dummies in this chapter.

- *EMG-based electrical stimulation*: These machines ask for some sort of effort before the electrical stimulation is sent into the muscles. Here's how it works: There is either a sound or a visual cue to open the hand. The survivor attempts to move the muscle. Once the muscles contract, even slightly, stimulation opens the hand. These machines are sensitive, so they can pick up muscle activity even if you can't see movement in the hand. These machines include the Mentamove, Biomove, NeuroMove™, and Saebo MyoTrac Infiniti.

- *Electrical stimulation orthotic*: This orthotic is rigid plastic that forms perfectly around the forearm and provides the stimulation to the muscles that need it. This orthotic has an advantage over other forms of electrical stimulation—you can move the arm and hand around and do real-world activities. The only orthotic to provide this is the Bioness H200™.

- *Spring-loaded finger extension orthotic*: This orthotic uses springs and pulleys attached to a rigid orthotic to facilitate opening the fingers. You can move the arm and hand around and do real-world activities while you perform grasping activities. The orthotic helps the fingers "release" once objects are grasped. The only orthotic to provide this is the SaeboFlex®.

Some of the machines suggested require specially trained therapists. In some cases, contacting the manufacturer is the best way to find therapists in your area who are using these machines. See Chapter 9: Recovery Machines for more information on all of the machines reviewed here.

All these machines have the potential of providing a small amount of voluntary movement. Once there is voluntary movement you can start doing repetitive practice on your own.

Here are three other ideas to help develop movement in the hand that do not involve machines.

- *Passively moving the joints*: Recent research has revealed that passively moving a joint will begin to slightly rewire the brain. This may provide a small spark to begin the neuroplastic process. Much more neuroplastic change will happen when you initiate the movement yourself, but for low-level stroke survivors, passively moving the joint may help. It is interesting to note that many of the robots used for rehabilitation, including the products made by Myomo™ (www.myomo.com), use *some* passive movement to promote recovery. These robots only help where help is needed, however. The more movement that you can do yourself, the more recovery you will get.

- *Repetitive practice into flexion*: Although it may not seem to make sense at first glance, tightening your fingers into a fist may help to gain control over your hand. The reason that stroke survivors have a hard time opening the hand is spasticity in the muscles that close the hand and fingers. As discussed in the section Neuroplastic Beats Spastic (see Chapter 7), spasticity is caused by too much spinal cord control and not enough brain control. Squeezing the hand will work the muscles to help re-establish brain control over those muscles. This will lead to less spasticity. If you choose this strategy, also work on relaxing the hand: You would first squeeze and then relax, squeeze, relax. To keep the fingernails from biting into the palm and also to practice this in different hand postures, squeeze an object. The classic example is a tennis ball. You can also use any number of squeeze toys or anything that will passively open the hand so you can make the next attempt at gripping the object. Mix *repetitive practice into flexion* with a robust stretching program. The fingers should be stretched into the most possible nonpainful extension of both the fingers and wrist at the same time ("prayer position").

- Mirror therapy (discussed fully in the section entitled Mirror Therapy later in this chapter) has been shown in some studies to jump start the neuroplastic process in lower-level stroke survivors. Mirror therapy involves observing the "good" side in a mirror so that the "bad" side looks like it's moving perfectly well. This therapy can be done even when there is little to no movement in the "bad" arm and hand.

So that continuum would be this: Use something (a machine, technique, etc., as outlined previously) to get just a little bit of movement. Use that movement repetitively. Once repetitive practice provides enough movement, you can use constraint-induced therapy (CIT) to take you the rest of the way.

What Precautions Should Be Taken?

Any sort of repetitive practice takes a lot of effort. You are working your muscles and your brain in ways that are "new" (new since the stroke). Both your muscles and your brain are changing. This change requires a lot of energy. Fatigue can cause less focus on safety. Less focus on safety can lead to injury, and injury can stop recovery. Be sure you are well rested.

IMAGINE IT!

Athletes do it. Musicians do it. Just about every motivational speaker recommends doing it. "It" is **mental practice** (MP)—also known as **imagery**. It has been used since the beginning of humankind to imagine an event before the event happens. This gives humans the unique ability to "practice" a task before it takes place. Although MP is done without actually moving, research has found that mental practice is *not* a passive process.

Mental practice, used alternately with actual practice, is an effective tool for recovery from stroke. It has the advantage of being easy, inexpensive, and safe, and it can be done almost anywhere.

Mental practice is actually an active process because:

- When you imagine moving your body, the muscles involved in those movements actually flex slightly, in exactly the same pattern they do during the actual movement.

- When you move you use a particular portion of your brain to do those movements. When you do MP of those same movements, the same areas in the brain are used.

- Mental practice has been shown to rewire the brain after stroke. Studies have shown that, in certain circumstances, mentally practicing something promotes as much neuroplastic change as actually practicing it!

- Mental practice is an active mental repetition of the task. Mental practice represents repeated attempts to imagine moving as one did prior to the stroke. Mental practice involves active, disciplined, and focused "mental attempts."

Immersive virtual reality (VR) has been shown to aid recovery after stroke (see You Are Game—Virtual Reality, later in this chapter). Immersive VR involves a "wrap-around" experience; wherever you turn your head, the virtual (artificial) environment is there. Mental practice resembles VR, but uses your mind instead of technology.

How Is It Done?

Mental practice has two elements to it:

- *Practicing the movement mentally*: Whatever movement you are actually physically practicing, that's what should be mentally practiced. So, if you are working on actually walking, support that actual practice with mental practice. Mental practice does not work well when there is no concurrent actual practice. The first thing to do is make an audio recording. The recording should first take you through a period of deep relaxation. The main idea during relaxation is to make yourself comfortable, empty the mind, and control breathing. The deep relaxation part of the tape should last three to five minutes. Following deep relaxation is the actual mental practice portion of the recording. This portion will describe the task that will be mentally practiced. The recording should involve every aspect of the experience, including the size of the room and full description of the movement, as well as the feel of the movement. It should sound something like, "Imagine you are sitting in your favorite chair. The room is quiet. There is a table in front of the chair. . . ." Later, the details of the movement are filled in: ". . . Imagine there is a glass on that table with fresh apple juice in it. Feel yourself reaching for the glass. Feel the weight of your arm as you reach out. Feel your elbow straightening and your wrist extending. Your hand opens, and your fingertips touch the cool glass . . ." and so on.

  It may be possible to do mental practice without the aid of an audio recording, but this has not been tested in research. Certainly athletes, musicians, and other performers use mental practice without audio recordings, so it may merit a try for stroke survivors as well. Just proceed through deep relaxation and then picture the movement. The more realistically you can imagine the task, the more effective the mental practice will be.

- *Practicing the movement in the real world*: Once the audio recording has been listened to a few times, practice the movement in reality. The ratio should be approximately three listening sessions to one actual practice session.

- When you are receiving therapy (occupational, physical, or speech therapy), mental practice can be used as an adjunct to actual practice. You can "expand the therapeutic footprint" by mentally practicing whatever you physically practiced in therapy. The "downtime" between therapy sessions can be used to magnify the positive effect of therapy with mental practice. (See the section Expanding the Therapeutic Footprint in Chapter 6, for more ideas on how to amplify the effect of therapy on your own.)

Again, please note: It is not necessary for you to have an audio recording to do mental practice. Let's say you are relearning to walk after stroke (called gait training). You can magnify gait training by going back to your room, relaxing, closing your eyes, and remembering how it felt to walk prior to your stroke. Try to make what you imagine as pristine as possible. That is, imagine walking down the street or path you know well. This will help you to clearly visualize walking as you did prior to the stroke.

What Precautions Should Be Taken?

Just because it is mentally practiced "perfectly" does not mean it can actually be done perfectly. The reality is that the stroke survivor may or may not move better after mental practice. Therefore, if the stroke survivor is attempting to walk, it is necessary to understand the difference between the perfect movements imagined during mental practice sessions and the real-world realities of gravity, effort, and endurance.

ELECTRICAL STIMULATION FOR FRUGAL DUMMIES

Let's say you wanted to do electrical stimulation (e-stim) to help your recovery. But there are two things stopping you:

1. You don't know what to do

2. E-stim is really expensive

Here's some good news: E-stim is easy and cheap.

How Is It Done?

There are three parts to any e-stim setup:

1. Machine   2. Lead wires   3. Electrodes

Put electrodes (they're usually sticky) over the muscle you want to work. Typically after stroke there are two sets of muscles that everyone focuses on:

The finger and wrist extensors; these will pull the wrist up and open the fingers.

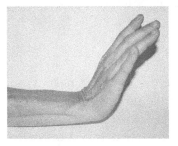

The muscles that lift the foot and end drop foot.

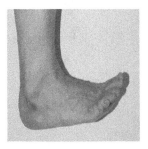

So, where do the electrodes go again?

Wrist/fingers:

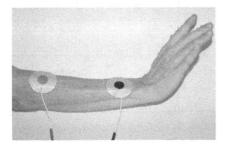

The muscles that lift the foot:

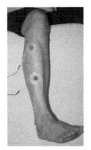

1. Attach the lead wires from the machine to the electrodes.

2. Stick on the electrodes according to the images preceding. Optimal placement will vary from person to person because everyone's anatomy is different. And, after stroke, every survivor's deficit will require slight changes in electrode placement according to their needs.

3. Turn up the e-stim. If you are getting the movement you want, take a photo of the electrode placement, or put a pen mark on your skin.

How long should I do it for? There have been a lot of "dosing" clinical trials for e-stim. Figuring dosing for e-stim is just what like figuring dosing for a drug:

- How much should I "take"? Is it different for every survivor? *Yes.*

- Does it depend on how much brain damage there was? *Yes.*

- Does it depend on other things as well? *Yes.*

The only way you'll learn how much e-stim you need and learn how to use the machine is to use the machine. Manuals and rules are nice, but practice is better. Put the electrodes on and turn up the e-stim slowly. Once you get the movement you want, note the amount of e-stim you used (measured in milliamps or mA). Two important notes:

1. **Make sure you gradate up the e-stim.** Basically, it's the same as any exercise program: Start slowly, and work up to more over time. Why gradate up? When e-stim is used and there is muscle contraction, that muscle is being worked. It is firing. Just like with any muscle work, you can end up sore and worse if you do too much too soon. So gradate up something like this:

   - Day 1: Two minutes
   - Day 2: Four minutes
   - Day 3: Six minutes
   - Day 4: Ten minutes
   - Day 5: Five minutes twice a day
   - Day 6: Eight minutes twice a day
   - Day 7: Ten minutes twice a day

And so on . . . until you hit the optimal dose and then stay there. This will give your muscles time to build gradually. If you get sore, reduce the dose.

1. *Make sure you ramp up the e-stim.* When E-stim makes your muscle fire it does not just affect *that* muscle. It also affects that muscle's antagonist (the muscle that moves in the opposite direction). An example is the elbow flexors (benders) and extensors (straighteners). If you e-stim the muscles that straighten the elbow, if done properly, the muscles that bend the elbow will be forced to relax. In most survivors where the elbow is always bent, it would be good (great!) to relax the muscles that bend the elbow. This phenomenon—when one muscle contracts, its opposing muscle relaxes—is called *reciprocal inhibition*. So that's good: You use e-stim to contract one muscle and relax the opposite muscle. But there is one problem . . .

If the highest amount of e-stim that is set happens all at once, a paradoxical thing happens. The muscle that should relax (the opposite or antagonist muscle), actually fires. It fires because it is trying to protect itself from being overstretched. So now both muscles are firing and essentially fighting each other.

To correct this, make sure the "ramp up time" is at least two seconds. The machine will let you control the amount of ramp up time. Make it two to five seconds; this will give the antagonist muscle time to not feel threatened and to relax.

So it will look something like this:

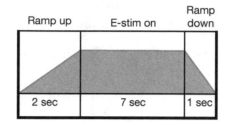

The cost is . . . cheap!

E-stim is inexpensive, and the web is a great place to start shopping. You're looking for NMES (**neuromuscular electrical stimulation**—where the muscle actually fires) not TENS (where you can feel it but the muscle does not fire).

What Precautions Should Be Taken?

Always consult your doctor when adding e-stim to your recovery plan. Some e-stim requires a doctor's prescription. Recovery options that involve e-stim have serious precautions and contraindications. Discuss these with your medical doctor prior to using any e-stim. Here is a partial list of contraindications and precautions for recovery options that use e-stim:

- Pregnancy
- Skin irritation
- Epilepsy/seizures
- Sensitive skin
- Compromised sensation
- Heart disease
- Pacemakers or defibrillators
- Recent surgery if muscle contraction may disrupt healing
- Electrode placement over the carotid sinus in the neck
- Existing thrombosis

STIMULATE YOUR STRIDE

Stroke survivors often have difficulty lifting their foot at the ankle (**dorsiflexion**). This problem is called "drop foot" or "foot drop." Foot drop leads to what is essentially an ongoing series of trips unless a style of walking is used that raises the leg enough to have the foot safely clear the floor. There are four types of walking patterns stroke survivors typically use when they have foot drop:

- *Steppage gait* involves lifting the foot high off the ground by overly bending the knee and hip.

- *Circumduction* involves sweeping the "bad" leg way out to the side so the foot can swing by.

- *Vaulting* involves raising the heel on the "good" leg in order to swing the affected leg through.

- *Hip hiking* involves lifting the "bad" leg by using the muscles in the trunk to "hike" the pelvis upward on the "bad" side. This allows the "bad" leg to swing through.

All of these styles of gait may bring a stroke survivor safely from point A to B. There is a downside to these sorts of unnatural walking patterns, however. Bone, cartilage, ligaments, and tendons work best during normal walking. The walking patterns often used after stroke cause stress on joints, the trunk, and back, which lead to arthritis and other disorders over time. Also, these altered forms of walking expend a lot more energy than "normal" walking. Most importantly, drop foot causes a gait that has the potential to lead to falls.

Doctors will prescribe an **ankle/foot orthosis (AFO)** for most stroke survivors who have drop foot. There are good reasons to wear AFOs; they:

- Lift the foot so that the survivor does not trip and the leg swings forward more naturally

- Stabilize the ankle so it does not twist—a twisted ankle can lead to a fall

- Allow walking to be safer

- Make walking take less energy, so you can walk farther

However, there is a downside to using AFOs. An AFO is used every day and, usually, for the rest of your life. Because the AFO lifts the foot, you will never need to lift your foot again. Once the AFO is consistently used, several things can happen to the brain and muscles that can eliminate the chance of ever walking without an AFO again. Use of an AFO:

- Weakens the muscles that are normally used to lift the foot

- Reduces the amount of brain dedicated to lifting the foot (learned non-use). A sort of reverse **neuroplasticity** occurs in the brain, so that the stroke survivor eventually loses any ability (or any future ability) to lift the foot on his or her own

- Reduces **passive range of motion**. The ankle is rarely taken through its full natural range of motion because the AFO inhibits normal movement. The soft tissue surrounding the joints shortens, and passive range of motion is lost.

You can "jump start" the process of lifting your foot on your own again, however. There are special functional electrical stimulation (FES) systems that can reverse the bad trends initiated by AFOs. These FES systems increase quality of movement, range of motion, and strength, and make walking safe and efficient. Research has shown that FES improves overall movement in the leg and improves walking ability.

How Is It Done?

There are muscles at the front of the lower leg, just to the outside of the shin bone, that lift the foot. These are the muscles that, when weakened by stroke, cause drop foot. FES systems provide low levels of electrical stimulation to the muscles that lift the foot while walking. Unlike an AFO, FES allows the stroke survivor's own muscles to do the work of lifting the foot. The stimulation is sent from a machine, either down a wire or through radio signals, into an electrode that lies against the skin, just over the muscles and nerves that lift the foot. A doctor or therapist adjusts the system to obtain the best foot movement for the highest quality of walking.

Companies that make FES systems for walking include (in no particular order) are NESS L300™ and the WalkAide® System. These devices are outlined, with websites included, in Chapter 9: Recovery Machines.

Functional electrical stimulation for walking may have more benefits than just helping you walk better. These systems may also:

- Strengthen muscles that are weak or paralyzed

- Stretch spastic muscles and other **soft tissue**

- Reduce spasticity
- Increase active range of motion
- Increase the amount of brainpower dedicated to lifting the foot
- Reduce falls

There is no sugar coating this one: These systems are expensive. We can assume that the cost will steadily decrease because of competition and other market forces.

What Precautions Should Be Taken?

This is not an off-the-shelf treatment. These systems require a prescription from a doctor and have to be fitted by a doctor or therapist. The stroke survivor needs specific training to start the therapy. The healthcare workers involved in the process will detail all the necessary precautions. Many questions ("Is this system appropriate for me?" "Is there a rental option or do you sell used machines?" "Who in my area is trained in this technology?") are often best answered by the vendors themselves. These vendors all have a website with a phone number.

MIRROR THERAPY (MT)

Please note: In this section, the word "limb" will be used for either the hand and/or arm or the foot and/or leg.

During **mirror therapy** (MT) you use a mirror to look directly at your "good" limbs. At the same time, your "bad" limbs are out of view, hidden behind a mirror. What you see looks a lot like both limbs moving perfectly well. But it's an illusion. What you are actually seeing is your good limb twice. One, of course, is your real limb; the other image is the reflection of your "good" limb. The reflection of your "good" limb makes it appear that both limbs are moving normally. Some research indicates that seeing the reflection of the "good" limb tricks the brain into believing the "bad" limb is moving perfectly well. The mirror provides proper visual input so the brain can "remember" how the "bad" limbs *should* move.

Most of the **neuroplastic** change outlined in this book involves rewiring the area of the brain that controls movement. MT may rewire both (1) the area that of the brain that controls sensation, and (2) the area of the brain that controls movement. MT may help make a visual connection to muscle control. This may strengthen the sensory-motor (feeling-moving) connection between muscle and the brain. MT has a motivating and encouraging quality. It is believed that the mirror encourages the survivor because the "bad" arm looks like it is moving correctly.

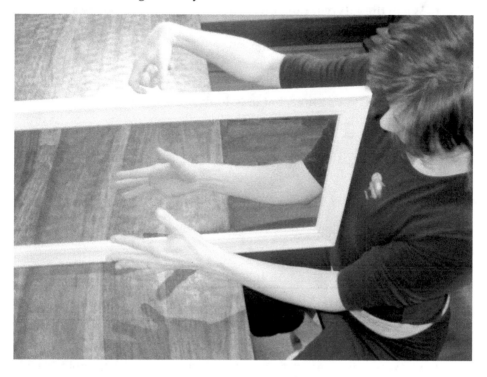

Brain scanning during MT has shown something rather curious. Even though the "good" limb is doing most of the work during MT, it is the "bad" side of the brain that is active. The illusion created by the mirror is so complete that it fools the injured side of the brain into working. And this phenomenon is seen even in low-level stroke survivors who cannot yet move their bad" limb.

How Is It Done?

You can use any sturdy and stable mirror to do MT. To set up: Sit with the mirror facing the "good" side of your body. Look at the reflection of the "good" limb and make sure you cannot see the "bad" limb. When you look in the mirror you will only see the "good" limb.

MT can be used at any point in recovery:

- **Before the survivor is able to move**: The survivor moves the "good" limb and observes it moving in the mirror. The "bad" limb does not move at all. MT can be in this way before the survivor can move the "bad" limb.

- **When the survivor can move**: Both sides are moved at the same time. The "bad" limb attempts to make the same movement as the "good" limb. The movements are done with both limbs at the same time. As much as possible the "bad" hand attempts to copy what the "good" hand is doing. Both hands are moved in the same way (symmetrically) at the same time, but only look at the "good" limb. The movements should be as equal as possible, like conducting an orchestra.

The movements attempted should be basic and may include . . .

Arm/hand:

1. Opening and closing the hand
2. Flipping the forearm and hand from palm down to palm up
3. Bending and straightening the wrist
4. Touching the thumb to the fingertips

Two things that you should keep in mind when deciding what movements to work on:

1. Work on movement that is on the edge of your ability. For instance, let's say you cannot yet open your hand but when you relax your hand it naturally falls open. Opening your hand is on the edge of your ability. Use hand opening on the "good" side while viewing it in the mirror.

2. As you gain ability, work bilaterally. That is, when your "bad" arm and hand get better movement, attempt to copy the "good" side movement. You'll be looking at the mirror, so it will look like you're doing it perfectly well (the mirror image of the "good" arm/hand). While you're actually moving the "bad" arm/hand—and maybe not even very well—you are viewing only the good movement. This bilateral work should only be attempted once the "bad" side is able to reasonably copy what the "good" side is doing.

MT can be done for the leg as well. It is usually done with the survivor sitting in a chair. The mirror is positioned between the two legs and the head is positioned on the side of the mirror that reflects the "good" leg. The survivor then looks at the mirror, which provides the reflection of the "good" leg. Two movements are usually the focus of lower extremity mirror therapy:

Foot/leg

1. Moving the foot up and down at the ankle (dorsiflexion).
2. Sliding the foot forward and backward (toward you). To make the sliding easier, wear a sock on a hard floor, or place a cloth under the foot.

In both the upper and lower limbs, the amount of mirror therapy that has been tested is 30 minutes per day. Typically the dosage will look something like this:

30 min 5 days a week for 4 weeks

2x daily 30 min; 2 days/week for 5 weeks

2x daily for 15 min; 6 days/week for 4 weeks

As is true with many treatment options for stroke, the exact dosage has not yet been determined. Therapists can help you figure out how long to do mirror therapy, and what movements should be practiced.

Note: Mirror therapy has been shown to reduce pain associated with shoulder-hand syndrome (SHS). Reduction of pain is achieved with exactly the same use of MT as outlined. A full explanation of SHS is available in the glossary.

What Precautions Should Be Taken?

Mirror therapy should be done in the seated position. Foot/leg mirror therapy may be done with the legs and feet while lying down or seated. Make sure that the mirror is stable so there is no risk of breakage.

RECOVERY OF FEELING

Human beings are great athletes. What makes us really special athletes is the ability to practice things repetitively. Although other animals practice skills repetitively, they tend to practice a very small set of survival skills. We can practice anything from throwing to climbing, and from tennis to kickboxing. We have another advantage: We, not instinct, determine the amount we practice. Animals also will only practice to the point in which they are good enough to use the skill to survive. We practice to the point of excellence.

Whenever we practice something we don't just practice the movement, we also practice the feeling of the movement. The *feeling* of movement (sensation) is essential to quality movement itself. Without the ability to feel, the movement becomes uncoordinated. In fact, the main reason we have sensation is to guide our movement.

In stroke survivors, the following is usually true:

- When sensation improves, movement usually improves.
- When movement is improved, sensation often recovers.

Sensation recovery involves the same rules of neuroplasticity as recovery of movement. The recovery of movement and sensation requires the same thing: **repetitive and demanding practice**. That is, if you feel something over and over and over, the portion of the brain that listens to that feeling expands. If a sensation is delivered repeatedly, over time that sensation is "felt" by the brain more strongly. Sensation follows the same rules of neuroplasticity as movement. What works to recover movement also works to recover sensation, and this is good news. You don't have to learn a completely new set of ideas in order to improve sensation.

It should be pointed out that researchers know a lot less about recovery of sensation than they know about recovery of movement. This is true for two reasons:

- There is a belief that recovery of movement is more important than recovery of sensation. Recovery of movement is what everybody wants. Therapists want it, stroke survivors want it, and insurance companies want it. Of course, everyone wants recovery of sensation, as well. Sensation is the Ying to movement's Yang; neither does well in isolation. But in the clinic, the focus is almost always on recovery of movement, not sensation.

- Recovery of movement is easy to see and measure. But recovery of sensation is impossible to observe and difficult to measure. You can see if somebody is moving better, but how do you tell if they're feeling more? It's a lot easier to treat what you can test than to treat what you can't observe.

There are two forms of sensation that most impact stroke recovery:

- **Proprioception**: The ability to know where parts of your body are without looking at them. Proprioception is essential to normal movement.

Some stroke survivors have great movement, but because they have poor proprioception, they don't move well. Lack of proprioception is called **apraxia**.

- **Tactile sensation**: The feeling of pressure on the skin; the sense of touch.

How Is It Done?

Repetitive practice of a movement makes that movement better. Repetitive practice works because every time you attempt to make a movement, the area in the brain that controls movement gets bigger. That's the essence of neuroplasticity: Whatever it is that you do repetitively changes the brain. The same is true for recovery of sensation. Repetitive *feeling* helps re-establish sensation. But movement and sensation depend on each other. In fact, the representation in the brain of movement and sensation are very close to each other. Both reside from about the crest of the ear to the top of the skull. And both are somewhat intertwined. They are so intertwined that every time you relearn a movement, you relearn sensation. This is a common theme often lost on doctors and even some therapists: Movement is good, even if the movement is not functional or necessary or pretty. Movement helps retrain movement, and it also helps retrain the sensation of movement (proprioception). So one way of recovering sensation you already know if you have read this far in the book: **constraint-induced therapy** (CIT). CIT involves many repetitions of movements. It also involves using the "bad" side limb during the many hours when the survivor is not in the clinic. CIT is believed to improve proprioception. Every time you move, the feeling of that movement is felt. That is, movement itself seems to drive increases in sensation. In reality, movement and sensation are two parts of the same thing. The more you move, the more the sensation of movement becomes ingrained into the neurons of the brain.

But what if you want to focus only on recovery of sensation. That is, what if you want to work on sensation more than just as a by-product of movement? If this is your goal, you have to "exercise" the sensation part of the brain. Efforts specific to sensation recovery involve two broad strategies:

- Passive: The survivor tries to feel something that's happening to them.
- Active: The survivor tries to feel something and then report what he or she feels.

Passive Training of Sensation (PTS)

Passive training of sensation (PTS) involves some tool that does something to the survivor. The survivor then attempts to feel what the tool is doing. The most common PTS involves electrical stimulation (e-stim). On the "good" side, stroke survivors can feel e-stim when it's turned up a little bit (typically around five milliamps). Of course, if you were to move those electrodes over to the "bad" side, the survivor with sensation loss would not be able to feel the e-stim. And that's exactly how e-stim is used to help recover sensation: The e-stim is turned up to just below where the survivor can feel it. They are then given a chance to sit quietly, often with their eyes closed, while trying to feel the "tap, tap, tap" that e-stim would normally deliver. Once they can feel that, they are "challenged" by having the e-stim turned down. If things go well, the e-stim can be turned down to close to the same level as the "good" side.

When you talk to your therapist about this, you can explain it easily by saying "TENS on the affected side." TENS is a term that therapists know well. It stands for transcutaneous *electrical* nerve *stimulation.* This sort of electrical stimulation is typically given for reduction of pain. However, it can also be used to retrain sensation after stroke.

The amount of time for which this treatment should be used is different for every survivor. Researchers have used single sessions of long duration. They also use multiple sessions spanning a long period of time (i.e., 30 minutes applied five days a week for eight weeks). Work with your therapist to figure out the right dosage for you. Note that e-stim does have some contraindications, so work with your healthcare professional to stay safe. However, once the proper treatment is determined, e-stim can often be used safely at home, and e-stim machines are relatively inexpensive (approximately $40).

There are other PTS treatments that have been used to help recover sensation, including . . .

- Pneumatic compression (a machine gently and repeatedly squeezes a limb on the affected side)
- Thermal stimulation (hot pack and cold pack, repeatedly)
- Vibration (a machine the gently vibrates a part of the body)

Massage can be helpful, as well. Massage repeatedly sends messages to the brain. This will expand the area of the brain that listens to those messages. With regard to massage, there is a very interesting phenomenon with some survivors. Some survivors can feel it when they massage themselves, but can't feel it when others do it. In this way, self-massage may help retrain sensation.

Active Training of Sensation (ATS)

Active training of sensation (ATS) involves having the stroke survivor continuously report what he or she is feeling. The following are some examples of ATS. All of the following involve two people: The stroke survivor and a helper (clinician, caregiver, etc.).

- *Localization:* The stroke survivor closes her eyes. The helper touches the survivor on the "bad" arm/hand or leg/foot. The survivor then puts her "good" side finger where she was touched.

- *Graphesthesia*: The stroke survivor closes his eyes. The helper uses the tip of a paperclip to draw simple designs on the "bad" arm/hand or leg/foot. The survivor then opens his eyes and attempts to draw the design with a pen.

- *Stereognosis*: The helper places common objects (e.g., walnut, marble, feather, shells, teaspoon, button, ring, coin, key) in the survivor's affected hand. The survivor tries to identify the object.

Recovery of proprioception (the feeling of movement) is important because it is difficult to move if you can feel the movement. Here is an example of a technique designed to retrain proprioception:

- *Proprioception*: The stroke survivor closes her eyes. The helper places and holds the "bad" arm/hand in a random position. With the eyes remaining closed, the survivor attempts to copy the position of the "bad" arm/hand with the "good" arm/hand. The survivor then opens the eyes and notes the position of both the "good" and "bad" side. This process is repeated. If things go well, the survivor begins to accurately copy where their "good" limbs are with their "bad" limbs.

The approximate dosage from research for active training of sensation is a few minutes per day of each task (localization, stereognosis, proprioception, etc.) over 30 treatment sessions.

SENSATION TYPE	WHAT THE HELPER DOES	WHAT THE SURVIVOR DOES
Localization "Where am I being touched?" 	Touches the survivor lightly on some part of their body on the affected side.	Touch—with the "good" side—the same spot the "bad" side was touched.
Graphesthesia "What shape is being traced on my skin?" 	Lightly traces a shape on the skin on some part of the body on the affected side.	Guess (or draw with the "good" hand) the same shape that was traced on the "bad" side.

SENSATION TYPE	WHAT THE HELPER DOES	WHAT THE SURVIVOR DOES
Kinesthesia 	Places and holds the "bad" side in a position.	Attempts to match the static position of the "bad" side with the "good" side.

(continued)

SENSATION TYPE	WHAT THE HELPER DOES	WHAT THE SURVIVOR DOES
	Moves the "bad" side	Attempts to match the movement of the "bad" side with the "good" side.

What Precautions Should Be Taken?

The forms of passive training of sensation (PTS) discussed previously require oversight by the appropriate healthcare provider. For example, both e-stim and hot/cold packs have the potential to seriously injure.

SPEAK MUSICALLY

The left side of the brain contains the language centers. Stroke on the left side of the brain may cause **aphasia** (trouble speaking or understanding what others are saying).

What if another area of the brain could take over for the damaged language portion of the brain? For instance, what if you could use a part of the *right* side of your brain for language? That is the aim of a therapy called **melodic intonation therapy (MIT)**. This therapy uses a person's innate ability to process music in retraining the ability to speak after stroke. The right side of the brain is where music is perceived.

It is remarkable to hear someone who can barely talk, sing beautifully, with diction and word-finding in full bloom. This ability to use the intact "music portion" of the brain to communicate is one of the bright spots in emerging research on rehabilitation from aphasia. MIT may be able to jump start the ability of the brain to rewire itself **neuroplastically**.

How Is It Done?

A speech therapist takes the stroke survivor through the process of retraining speech using MIT. This therapy may be effective in stroke survivors with certain deficits but who also have particular strengths. For instance, the best candidates for MIT are folks who:

- Can presently speak very little
- Can process sound correctly
- Understand when they make mistakes
- Are able to correct mistakes
- Are emotionally stable

MIT involves exaggerating the sing-song aspect of speech. The stroke survivor is encouraged to express language as a series of tones, allowing words to form notes, and sentences to form melody. Imagine the song-like quality of children as they memorize a nursery rhyme, repeat their ABCs, or learn to count. This is much the same technique used to emphasize the pitch and rhythm of language. This may stimulate the right side of the brain to provide some of the power needed to speak.

What Precautions Should Be Taken?

This therapy is done under the supervision of a speech therapist.

CONSTRAINT-INDUCED THERAPY FOR SPEECH

Constraint-induced therapy (CIT) in the arm and leg involves focusing the entire treatment on the "bad" side. In the upper extremity, the "good" arm and hand is constrained, usually with a sling or a mitt. This makes CIT in the arms relatively straightforward. In the leg, there is a problem, because if you tie up the "good" leg, you're asking for trouble! Therapists handle the challenge of using CIT in the leg by overloading the leg with large amounts of safe exercises. CIT for **expressive aphasia**, called constraint-induced aphasia therapy (CIAT), shares many of the same techniques used in arms and legs.

How Is It Done?

All of the constraint therapies require:

- *Hours per day of focused and dedicated practice* for approximately two to three weeks

  — CIT: Between five and seven hours a day of movement practice

  — CIAT: Delivered with schedules of two to three hours a day. Research indicates that this level of intensity is necessary to rewire the language areas of the brain

- *Forcing the stroke survivors to work on their weakness*

  — CIT: Uses a sling or mitt to constrain the "good" hand

  — CIAT: Prevents nonverbal communication, including hand gestures, writing, and drawing

- *Repetition of desired behavior*

  — CIT: Movements are practiced over and over

  — CIAT: Sounds, words, and sentences are repeated

- *Constant challenge*

  — CIT: Movements attempted are made difficult over time

  — CIAT: More difficult sounds, words, and sentence structures are attempted over time

For better speech to occur, intense, focused, and repeated attempts have to be made. This will provide new pathways for neurons (nerve cells) in the brain. These pathways become stronger with each repetition and end up "hard wiring" to each other, allowing the stroke survivor to speak better.

In some ways, CIAT is designed to do exactly the opposite of what stroke survivors with aphasia tend to do naturally. Here are some examples:

- Folks who are aphasic tend to not speak much because they feel that communicating may not be worth the effort. They often simply stop trying to talk at all or give up in the middle of sentences. CIAT does not allow *not* talking, or abandoning what you want to say. In fact, it forces hours of speaking a day.

- Folks who are aphasic tend to use other forms of communication, like gesturing, tone of voice on a single repeated word, or writing.

This is where the constraint part of CIAT comes in. During CIAT you are not allowed to communicate in any way that does not involve talking.

CIAT is done under the supervision of a speech therapist. Constraint therapies tend to be expensive because of the large number of clinical hours involved. Insurance does not typically pay for CIT or CIAT. Of course, just like many of the ideas in this book, certain elements of CIAT can be done on your own. There are elements of all the constraint therapies, including CIAT, that you can adopt and make part of your recovery effort. Repetition of sounds, words, and sentences and focused, dedicated practice can be done at home to augment what you learn with your speech therapist.

What Precautions Should Be Taken?

Consult your doctor prior to starting this therapy. CIAT is nothing if not vigorous, and the implications of the effort and frustrations inherent in relearning to talk may have global health implications.

YOU ARE GAME—VIRTUAL REALITY

Virtual reality (VR) has the potential to make recovery fun while being safe and challenging. You can become involved in the game either by wearing a VR mask or goggles, or by looking at a TV or computer screen. While playing, you are physically challenged. For instance, a game may ask the player to catch a virtual ball or use a plastic saber to slay characters on the screen. The great thing about VR is that you can challenge yourself in new and imaginative ways, safely seated in the most comfortable chair in your home.

People love video games because they are designed to have an interesting and realistic look. They are fun, competitive, and challenging. Many people look at video games as passive entertainment. But for the stroke survivor, VR provides a physical challenge that has one strong advantage over real-world rehabilitation: *safety*. With video games, you can walk, run, and ski . . . perform almost any activity within the safety of an armchair. Stroke survivors can use VR to help develop better balance, better arm and hand movement, and increased strength. Unfortunately, much of stroke recovery can be boring. Many repetitions of a movement are needed to rewire the brain to make that movement better. But repeating a movement thousands of times is not the most interesting way to spend your time. This is especially true because, during recovery from stroke, you are not learning new and exciting skills. You are simply relearning skills that you did perfectly prior to your stroke. VR allows repetitive practice to occur while using your own natural sense of competition and creativity in an engaging environment. In short, VR makes repetitive practice fun.

How Is It Done?

VR gaming systems are available in toy stores for under $50. The fact that many of the games are inexpensive allows you to be creative while managing your own recovery. Use games that are challenging, fun, and maintain safety.

VR technology can be an effective way of increasing active movement in the hands and arms after stroke. The trick is finding a game that will challenge the hand and arm in a way that is interesting and fun. Therapies that engage you tend to be more productive, so make sure the game is interesting to you. Make sure the game challenges you in a way that promotes recovery. Using virtual reality as a recovery tool can be as simple as a joystick. For instance, if you decide that you need help with small amounts pronation (forearm palm down) and supination (forearm palm up), then a joystick might be the perfect recovery tool.

Many of these games are "plug and play" so that they plug right into your TV. However, VR that is immersive is more effective than games played on flat screens. Immersive means that you are wearing a head-mounted display or 3-D glasses. As you turn your head, you are completely surrounded by the visual experience.

The bottom line is that VR can help make motor learning after stroke fun. So indulge in the fun! When else are you, as an adult, allowed to play hours and hours of a video game and call it "work"?

What Precautions Should Be Taken?

VR may not be a safe option for balance exercises in some stroke survivors. However, leg exercises can be made safe by using your legs to play the game while you are sitting. For instance, if the game asks you to kick a ball, make sure you can accomplish this while sitting in a chair.

Just like any exercise, VR should be done within the recommendations of your doctor. Discontinue any exercise if it causes pain. Because VR is engaging, you might be less aware of discomfort or safety issues. It is prudent to consult with a therapist prior to using rehabilitation gaming so that the training is effective and safe.

THE GOOD TRAINS THE BAD—BILATERAL TRAINING

Most of the movements people do are **bilateral** (using either the arms/hands or the two legs working together). Even the movements that you think are done with just one limb involve the other limb without you even thinking about it. Consider handwriting. It turns out that the nonwriting hand has an important role in shifting the paper. Handwriting will get much slower and sloppier if the nonwriting hand is not involved. Another example is threading a needle. It would be easy to believe that if the needle was held steady in a vise that it would be easier to thread because the needle would be held perfectly stationary. Yet, when someone encounters this situation, the first instinct is to hold the needle. It turns out that when a person threads a needle, both hands are involved in an intricate and effective dance to get the needle threaded as efficiently as possible.

For folks who have *not* had a stroke, research has shown something remarkable. When both hands are used together in tasks, the movement of the nondominant hand (in most of us, the left hand) improves movement quality, accuracy, and speed. Researchers have found a similar dynamic in stroke survivors. When the "good" arm and "bad" arm are doing the same movements at the same time, the "bad" arm moves better. This is also true when the two arms do equal and opposite movements. When the two limbs are moved together, the movement in the affected limb improves its quality and accuracy. Using **bilateral training** helps the unaffected side train the affected side. In the leg, walking provides automatic bilateral training. Since you can't walk with one leg, the "bad" leg is forced to work, bilaterally, with the "good" leg. This may be one reason that the leg tends to recover faster than the arm. The arm and hand also benefit from this sort of training, but recovery efforts have to be specifically set up to allow for this type of training in the arm and hand.

This idea of having "the good side train the bad side" is appropriate for stroke survivors with limited available movement. This is one of the things that set bilateral training apart from other stroke recovery options. There are many repetitive practice options that work well with survivors who have "some" movement. For example, with some finger movement, more finger movement can be gained with repetitive practice.

There are few options for stroke survivors that have very limited amounts of movement. Bilateral training is appropriate for survivors with limited movement for two reasons:

1. Bilateral training in the arm and hand only requires a little available movement in the shoulders and elbows. Because recovery tends to be from proximal (close to the body) to distal (farther away from the body), bilateral training may initiate the process. The same is true for the lower extremity. Although the ankle may not yet be moving, bilateral training of the hip and knee may begin to promote ankle movement.

2. It is believed that bilateral training works because the two extremities communicate (one arm with the other and one leg with the other). And this communication is not through the brain—but through the spinal cord. The mechanism that allows this communication is believed to reside in the spinal cord and is known as the "central pattern generator" (CPG). The CPG is evident in many animals that exhibit rhythmic behavior. The CPG is the system that allows young infants to take "steps" suspended over the floor.

That the two limbs communicate with each other without the brain is good news for folks that have brain injury, like stroke. The "good" side training the "bad" side before the brain is involved is especially important for stroke survivors with very limited movement.

How Is It Done?

The best way to allow for bilateral training of the arm and hands is to promote movement where the two extremities do the same (or equal) but opposite movements. The arm will follow what the hand attempts, so the hand will be the primary focus in the following exercises.

Bilateral training can take two forms:

- *Equal and at the same time*: The two hands can work in unison (the same movement at the same time, as in a mirror image):
  — Throwing a two-handed basketball pass
  — Folding clothes symmetrically

— Pretending to conduct an orchestra to classical music

— Drumming both hands at the same time (add challenge by playing to music)

— Placing objects (blocks, cups, cones) close to you and then away from you at the same time

— Spooning out dry ingredients with both hands at the same time

- *Equal and alternating (reciprocal):* The two hands can work in equal opposition (each arm and hand does equal but opposite movements):

— Alternate punching

— Drumming

— Asymmetrical cloth folding

— Hand-.over-hand rope pulling

— Alternating wiping of a table with a towel

— Tapping a target while alternating hands

— Tapping a balloon from one hand to the other (add difficulty by tossing a ball from one hand to the other)

The possibilities are endless. All of these can be done to a rhythm (see the section Rhythm Rehab for the Arms and Hands later in this chapter), which will make you focus on equal movement done during equal amounts of time. The rhythm in music or the constant click of a metronome can be used to make the two limbs do the task within the same time limits.

All of the previously listed suggestions involve the arms and hands, but similar exercises can be performed with the legs and feet. With the leg and foot, the rules are the same as the arm and hand: Whatever movement one leg does, the other matches (equal and at the same time, and equal and alternating).

The more you match the movements of the "good" limb, the better. If you find matching the two limbs is too easy, add difficulty by adding speed. That is, accelerate the movement of the "good" limb, and try to continue to match the movement with the "bad" limb. Rhythmic movements with the legs and feet can be done while lying on the back, sitting, or in a recumbent position.

What Precautions Should Be Taken?

Most of these exercises can be done in a seated position with little or no significant risk. If any of these exercises are done in a standing position, added stress is put on balance, leg strength, and stamina. For this reason, do not perform this sort of bilateral training while standing without the recommendation of your doctor and the guidance of physical and/or occupational therapy staff.

RHYTHM REHAB FOR THE ARMS AND HANDS

It's a cliché that many people have heard: "Rhythm is essential to life." Much of what we do, from the grand cycles of life and death, to the pulse of heartbeats and the pattern of breathing, is rhythmic. There is power in rhythm that can be used to recover from stroke. Some aspects of recovery are naturally rhythmic. Walking and stationary cycling movements are rhythmic, but both are lower-extremity exercises. Setting up challenges that involve rhythm for the upper extremity requires a little creativity and ingenuity.

You need some sort of machine to provide a beat. This can be a metronome, which is a machine that musicians use to keep a constant rhythm. Inexpensive metronomes cost about $10. Most electronic keyboards, which usually have some sort of beat-keeping mechanism built in, can be used. Of course, the easiest way to involve a beat in recovery is listening to music. As long as the music has a constant beat, music will work. Music has an added advantage: It takes your mind off the fatigue factor. There is a reason that most exercise videos involve music: Listening to music provides a distraction from the difficulty of the exercise. This is the same reason that so many runners listen to music and the reason music headsets are banned from many running races. Because it mitigates pain, music is thought to provide an unfair advantage to athletes during strenuous athletic events.

Music may have the added benefit of providing motivation. Nothing motivates people like their favorite music. Music can become the soundtrack of your life that, just like in movies, adds color to recovery efforts.

How Is It Done?

Here is a simple way a beat can be used to help the "good" arm/hand to train the "bad" arm/hand:

- Place two towels on a table.

- Measure how far the "bad" hand can reach while sliding the towel across the table. Make sure the affected elbow is at its fullest extension

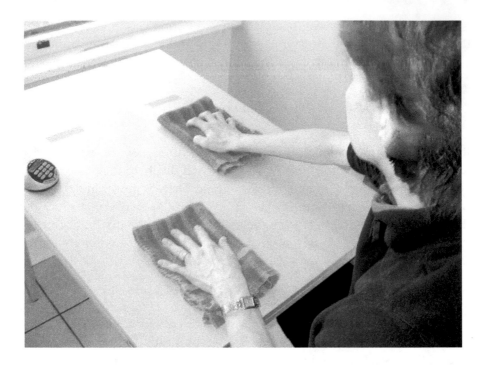

(most straight) and your back is against the seat back. Place a piece of tape at the furthest point you can reach, directly in front of the hand. Repeat the process for the "good" hand.

- Sit at the table so that one hand and wrist is on each towel. Keep your back against the seat back.

- Set the metronome so you can hit the targets on clicks. With each successive click, have your unaffected hand and then your affected hand push the towel forward until the tape target is met.

- Movement can be done in opposite: When one hand goes forward the other goes back. Or the movement can be done equally: Both hands go in the same direction at the same time.

- Increase the speed of the beat or the distance reached to increase challenge.

The same basic rules would apply to any exercise you devise. Simply follow these guidelines:

- The targets for each may be different, with each limb being asked to do what it can. For instance, the "good" limb may be asked to reach forward sixteen inches. The "bad" side limb may—depending where that limb is in the arc of recovery—only be asked to do five inches.

- Set a rhythmic rate that is slow and easy. This is not about going as fast as possible. This is about hitting the target on the beat.

- Set a timer so you know when to start and when to stop. If you use music, use the length of the song or piece as the start and stop points.

- Keep the rhythm!

What Precautions Should Be Taken?

Special emphasis should be placed on the possibility of spikes in blood pressure and pulse rate because this type of therapy can increase both.

For the upper extremities, this is a relatively safe technique, but again, if used for walking, marching, or anything that involves balance, be extra cautious, and consult your physician and physical therapist.

WALKING IN RHYTHM

Physical therapists focus on the mechanics of gait (how the legs and feet are used during walking). There is another important aspect to walking that gets less attention: rhythm. Walking after a stroke is often like bicycling on two square tires; there is a lack of a predictable rhythm. Researchers have successfully used what is called **rhythmic auditory cuing** to revive proper rhythm during walking. Any sort of rhythmic movement in the legs, arms, or a combination of all four limbs can benefit from this technique. This may even be worth a try with expressive aphasia. If words come out slowly, matching words to an increasing rhythm may accelerate the rate at which words can be formed. Using rhythm for recovery in the legs involves listening to and matching a beat while you walk. This can help re-establish the natural rhythm of gait. Developing a good and natural rhythm will help walking look and feel smoother and more symmetrical.

How Is It Done?

This sort of auditory cuing is simply a constant "click," like the ticking of a clock. In research experiments, a metronome (a device that musicians use to keep time while practicing their instruments) is used. Metronomes can be purchased for less than $10. There are many free metronome phone apps. Any device that produces a constant and predictable beat can be used. As long as the speed of the beat can be altered, a drum machine, a keyboard with programmable beats, or a metronome can be used. Music can be used, as well. The company Biodex has a treadmill specifically designed to provide audio feedback to encourage symmetry in walking. The company Interactive Metronome makes a product called the Gait Mate, which helps to re-establish rhythmicity by giving the survivor constant feedback. Sensors are put in the shoe under the heel, and those sensors tell the survivor, through headphones, when their foot is hitting the floor. This technology further attempts to re-establish rhythmicity by matching the survivor's footfalls against a constant beat. All this is done with real-time feedback to the survivor. (see Chapter 9: Recovery Machines).

However, simple technologies can be used as well. A metronome either heard through headphones or carried by the therapist as the survivor walks can be used to recover the rhythmicity of gait. Plugging the ears using standard noise-reducing plugs can boost the volume of footfalls to make them obvious to the survivor. The task is then to match the footfalls to the beat.

The trick is finding a constant rhythm that is close to the rhythm of comfortable walking. Researchers have often found it difficult to have patients match the beat of music precisely during walking. This therapy can be done while marching in place and while holding on to something strong, solid, and immobile. A wall-mounted bar or a sturdy chair may provide the necessary element of safety while marching in place. During treadmill walking, rhythm can be used to establish the rhythm of footfalls.

When the foot hits the ground (cadence) can be sped up or slowed down by changing the length of your steps. Shortening steps will speed up cadence, and lengthening steps will slow down cadence.

This concept of using rhythm to help the timing of movement may also help in other ways. Experiments have shown that people who run while listening to music feel less fatigue than those who don't listen to music. The same may be true with stroke survivors. Music can provide a hypnotic escape from an otherwise boring exercise routine.

What Precautions Should Be Taken?

The lower extremities of stroke survivors are notoriously hard to lock into a beat. The differences in strength and coordination between the "good" and "bad" sides make keeping a constant and steady beat while walking near impossible.

Even for folks who have not had a stroke, walking in perfect rhythm is difficult. There is a reason that the military spends so much time having soldiers walk in rhythm; it's hard to do. For this reason, the following recommendation exists:

Do not do this sort of rhythmic training while standing or walking without the recommendation of your doctor and the guidance of physical and/or occupational therapy staff.

SHOCKING SUBLUXATION

When someone has a stroke, there is often a period of time when the muscles on the affected side are completely limp (flaccid). During this stage of recovery, there is no muscle activity. Even basic reflexes that keep muscles tight (spastic) in later **stages of recovery** are not present. Muscles are usually flaccid right after the stroke, but flaccid muscles can continue for years. When the muscles that hold the shoulder joint in place are flaccid, the shoulder will often dislocate. In stroke survivors, shoulder dislocation is called **subluxation of the shoulder**.

The shoulder is an unusual joint. It is called a ball-in-socket joint, but should be called a "ball-on-a-flat-surface joint." Unlike other four-limbed animals, humans have developed forelimbs (arms) that have a huge **range of motion** at the shoulder. This gives us the ability to move our hands around in a wide area, which gives us the ability to do everything from throwing to climbing.

Humans pay a price for this great movement: The shoulder joint is relatively weak. The joint is formed by one round surface (the round top or "head" of the bone that makes up the upper arm) and a flat area, which is part of the shoulder blade. The shoulder joint is held together rather weakly by muscles that surround the joint. If these shoulder muscles become either weak or paralyzed, the weight of the arm pulls the joint apart. In some stroke survivors, the shoulder muscles reawaken as recovery continues, and the shoulder joint is pulled back into proper alignment. In other stroke survivors, shoulder subluxation can continue for years.

Along with the naturally weak human shoulder joint and the increased weakness of the joint after stroke, stroke survivors have an added risk: well-meaning people pulling on their affected arm. During transfers (e.g., sitting to standing, lying down to sitting) it is common for healthcare workers or caregivers to use the "bad" side arm to pull the stroke survivor into position. It "makes sense" to move the survivor in this way because the "bad" arm provides leverage for the weak side of the body. But resist the temptation to move a survivor with the arm if it puts pressure on the shoulder joint! Using the shoulder to move the survivor can cause permanent damage and pain to the shoulder.

When a muscle is completely flaccid after stroke, only one thing can make it contract: electrical stimulation (**e-stim**). This treatment is called **neuromuscular electrical stimulation (NMES)**. NMES involves sticky electrodes that are put on the skin over the target muscles. Wires go from the electrodes to the NMES machine. E-stim goes . . .

- From the machine to
- The wires to
- The electrodes to
- The skin and
- Into the muscles under the skin.

The e-stim can be turned up to the point where the muscle will contract. When using e-stim for shoulder subluxation (dislocation) after stroke, e-stim goes into the muscles that surround the shoulder joint.

When the stimulation enters the muscle, the muscle contracts and pulls the top arm bone (humerus) into proper position. The e-stim actually contracts (tightens) the muscles, in much the same way the stroke survivor would, if they could. E-stim can, over time, strengthen the muscles surrounding the shoulder joint. For some stroke survivors, this helps normal muscle activity hold the joint together permanently.

How Is It Done?

You'll need a clinician to determine the proper electrode placement for e-stim/dislocation. The following may be of more interest to clinicians than survivors:

There has been some debate about where electrodes should be placed for NMES and subluxation. Traditionally, the placement has been the deltoid and supraspinatus. However, it has been pointed out that the placement over the supraspinatus is problematic because the supraspinatus is covered by the upper trapezius. It is thus unlikely that the supraspinatus can be activated by surface stimulation. A better choice is the deltoid and the infraspinatus and teres minor.

Many machines on the market can provide electrical stimulation, in the proper dose, to resolve subluxation. A doctor's order and a therapist's guidance will establish the best electrode placement and type of stimulation parameters.

Percutaneous (performed through the skin) **intramuscular stimulation** (perc-NMES) is another option. This form of stimulation is much like NMES, but the electrodes are placed directly into the weakened muscles. This means that less e-stim is needed because there is less tissue between the machine and the muscles. Perc-NMES also has the advantage of being able to more accurately target the specific muscles that can help reduce subluxation. This treatment involves minor surgery.

Note that NMES is different from the form of e-stim that is often used clinically, called transcutaneous electrical nerve stimulation (TENS), often used to reduce pain, even the pain of subluxation. The TENS sort of e-stim does not make the muscle contract, and so would be ineffective in reducing subluxation.

What Precautions Should Be Taken?

Your doctor will let you know if this therapy will be effective and safe for you. There are some contraindications for e-stim because the electrical output can interfere with other electrical devices (e.g., pacemakers). Always consult your doctor before attempting this therapy. Have your occupational or physical therapist help you decide how and where the stimulation should be used. Once your doctor and therapist are consulted, e-stim may be able to be administered with an inexpensive machine, at home.

THE NEUROPLASTIC MODEL FOR "PUSHER" SYNDROME

Pusher syndrome (PS) is an altered sense of balance. Survivors with PS believe they're vertical (upright) when they are leaning toward the "bad" side. When they are forced upright by someone else (usually a therapist), they feel like they're leaning too far toward the "good" side. They see any attempt to get them truly vertical as a serious threat that inspires fear. "Pushers" react to this fear by "pushing" toward the "bad" side. Another term for pusher syndrome is *listing phenomenon*. This may be a more accurate term because "pushers" only become "pushers" when they are pushed. Anyone who was shoved out of balance would push back!

There are other terms that have been used for PS, including:

- Ipsilateral pushing
- Contraversive pushing
- Pusher behavior

Survivors with PS have damage to a portion of the brain that relays information about body posture from the body to the brain. The area damaged, near the middle of the brain, is called the posterolateral thalamus. When stroke damages this area, survivors can develop PS. PS affects approximately 5 percent of all stroke survivors. However, some estimates are as high as 50 percent.

How Is It Done?

Survivors with PS have trouble knowing when they're standing or sitting upright. In other words, they have trouble with balance. Balance is determined by three systems controlled by the brain:

1. Vision

2. Vestibular (inner ear)

3. Proprioception (feeling where your body is in space)

PS is damage to only one of the three systems: *proprioception*. Survivors with PS can retain balance by focusing on the systems that are still intact. Therapists help survivors develop strategies to overcome balance problems caused by PS. These strategies include focusing on vertical visual cues in the room. The idea is to use vision to overcome the lack of proprioception. The survivor is asked to reorient himself or herself to vertical. As is true with many of the recovery options that drive neuroplastic change, it is repeated *self*-correction that rewires the brain. Therapists will challenge survivors with PS by having them repeatedly reach for objects on the "bad" side. The survivor is then instructed to bring himself or herself back to vertical. This allows for neuroplastic rewiring of the brain through repetitive practice. The survivor is asked to repeatedly lean toward the "bad" side and then back to vertical. It is important that the survivor is in control of the attempts to come back to upright. Therapists can provide tricks and strategies to help the survivor move back to vertical. It is beneficial for survivors with PS to carry what they learned in the clinic to their everyday life. No matter what the activity, adjusting body posture to vertical will help survivors recover the ability to maintain proper balance.

What Precautions Should Be Taken?

Note that some research indicates that most survivors with PS spontaneously and completely regain their sense of balance within six months.

5 Elements of Exercise Essential to Recovery

HORIZONTAL REHAB: GOOD SLEEP = GOOD RECOVERY

One of the best things that you can do for your recovery is *get enough sleep*. Research in this area has been clear: *Sleep helps recovery*. Note that while enough sleep aids recovery, the opposite is true as well: *Not enough sleep hurts recovery*.

Studying how sleep affects recovery is simple. Researchers look at two groups of stroke survivors. One group gets plenty of sleep, and the other group has their sleep periodically disturbed. In both human and animal studies, the participants that get enough sleep recover more. Adequate sleep is beneficial to both mental and physical recovery. What you learn while you're awake (and this includes learning movement) is imprinted into the brain while you're sleeping. Sleep is not just a luxury; it is a vital part of recovery itself. Remember, stroke recovery requires **motor learning**. Motor learning, like any learning, involves making new connections between neurons in the brain. In this way, sleep is essential to moving better.

Stroke is brain damage. Brain damage caused by stroke can disrupt normal sleep cycles. Some survivors have found that periods of rest and/or regular naps can help. Some research has shown that naps actually lower the risk of dying of heart disease and stroke. The sleeping habits of humans were developed over hundreds of thousands of years of evolution. People are "programmed" to go to bed when the sun goes down and wake up as the sun rises. Artificial lighting, TVs, computers, and so on trick your brain into thinking it is daytime, even during the night. Going to bed at a set hour helps promote adequate sleep.

How Is It Done?

General suggestions for promoting adequate sleep:

- Close the sleeping room door
- Put a sign on the door and inform everyone that you're going to sleep
- Wear earplugs
- Use a "white noise" machine or fan to drown out outside noise
- Make the room dark. Light tricks the brain into believing it's daytime, even if it's 3 a.m. Turn off electronic devices. This includes TVs, computers, and so on. These devices, because they are lit, fool the brain into thinking that it's daytime
- Lower the room temperature. The best room temperature is about 65°F (18°C). Warm air fools the brain into believing it's daytime
- Physically (let it touch your skin) expose yourself to sunlight in the morning
- Be consistent with your schedule; get up and go to sleep at the same time every day
- Avoid electronic screens (TV, ebooks, phone) one to two hours before bedtime
- Exercise! Exercise promotes sleep

What Precautions Should Be Taken?

Sleep-aid drugs do not induce the same sort of learning benefit as natural sleep does. During natural sleep, the brain is very active. Natural sleep is when your brain consolidates new, important information while pitching unnecessary and redundant information. Natural sleep is active. Drugged sleep slows down brain activity.

Note that falling asleep, or dozing, during the daytime is actually an indicator for future strokes. People who fall asleep unintentionally have a four to five times greater risk of stroke than folks who don't doze.

GET A HOME EXERCISE PROGRAM

Being able to depend on physical, occupational, and speech therapists for ongoing therapy is an ideal situation. Therapists provide experience, knowledge, guidance, and encouragement. Unfortunately, therapists, and the facilities where therapists work, are expensive. Insurance will only pay for a certain amount of therapy. So what's a stroke survivor to do?

A home exercise program (HEP) is the group of exercises that the therapist gives you to do at home after all the therapy sessions are over. These exercises are usually given right before being discharged from therapy. The HEP may be provided before **discharge** from the hospital, again just before discharge from any skilled nursing facility, again during outpatient therapy, and then again at the end of any home therapy.

Therapists tend to leave the review of HEP until the final few visits, and the HEP usually is simply a rehash of the exercises done with the therapist during the course of therapy. Stroke survivors are handed a few photocopies of pictures or descriptions of exercises, and a review of those exercises is done. Here's a little a joke for this process:

"What does HEP stand for?"

"Hand 'Em Photocopies."

There are two problems with looking at the HEP in this "last-minute" way.

1. (*Before therapy has ended.*) The HEP should be started much, much earlier. In fact, the HEP can start during the acute phase and continue for the entire journey toward recovery. The HEP is more than just a bunch of exercises. It is a series of responsibilities that the survivor has to his or her own recovery. See the section Expanding the Therapeutic Footprint in Chapter 6 for a list of responsibilities that could easily become part of the HEP.

2. (*After therapy has ended.*) Making a lifelong plan toward recovery is essential to maximizing potential. Therapist-developed HEPs tend to be rigid, reflecting only what is on the photocopied pages. This casual

view is not only short-sighted, but it is actually detrimental to any further recovery. The traditional view of a HEP promotes the assumption that the stroke survivor won't get any better. This is a built-in, self-fulfilling prophecy. The same exercises that . . .

- . . . were used in therapy
- . . . did not promote progress toward the end of therapy
- . . . did achieve plateau
- . . . triggered the end of therapies
- will, at best, retain the present level of strength, coordination, and ability.

The thinking is, "Since the clinicians have determined that the survivor won't improve, they should keep doing the same thing to, at least, maintain the present level of recovery." This is true from a purely statistical standpoint; most patients either do not progress or actually get worse after discharge from therapy. Because of this thinking, the typical HEP has no built-in points at which it should be updated and no flexibility to help promote progress toward recovery. Keep in mind this thinking was influenced much more by managed care (insurance) than any philosophy that therapists have. There was a day in the United States, not too long ago, when therapists could spend much more time with stroke survivors. This allowed for more time to develop treatment plans like the HEP. In rehabilitation, this changed with the 1997 Balanced Budget Act. What was specifically implemented was called the prospective payment system (PPS). The PPS affected payments for rehab services and affected how long survivors can be seen in the following settings:

Inpatient rehabilitation hospitals

Skilled nursing facility services

Home health services

Hospital outpatient services

Outpatient rehabilitation services

The HEP is rushed because the system rushes. In any case, the view that you want more out of your HEP will be an unusual view to most therapists, so you may have to coach them through the process. For instance, perhaps you are not walking upon discharge from all therapies. But after you are discharged, you start a new leg strengthening program that allows you to take a few steps. What do you do now? How do you build on this progress? How do you develop the cardiovascular stamina to walk farther? Which muscles should you stretch, and which should you strengthen to facilitate more walking?

Let therapists know that what is required is a strategy that will help you to continue to make *gains*. Ask them to build into a HEP the flexibility that will constantly provide higher goals, and ask therapists to provide the tools and strategies to achieve those goals. These requests are going to challenge therapists in ways that they are not usually challenged, and you may get some strange looks. But therapists are highly trained and highly skilled in developing plans that promote recovery. Remember, you are paying (and paying well) for therapy, and having them provide an adequate and challenging HEP is well within their job description.

Also, challenge your physiatrist and therapists with suggestions of techniques and technologies that you find during your research. If you see something that you think would work, ask them to follow through by explaining and implementing that therapy. You were most likely discharged because these health professionals believed that you have **plateaued** (not going to get any better). If therapists just continue to use the same techniques then, indeed, you will not get any better. Why? Because, the same techniques will probably continue to get the same results. In your own attempts toward recovery, look for new therapies that might work, and have doctors and therapists implement the therapies.

How Is It Done?

A HEP that includes effective therapeutic interventions and exercises is essential to ongoing recovery from stroke. Here are some suggestions when consulting with a therapist about the HEP:

- Start planning your HEP with your therapists as early as possible. Tell all therapists—from the hospital to home therapy—to provide the information and tools needed to continue progress at home.
- Let therapists know that you want a strategy that will help you continue to make significant gains, not retain existing levels of performance.
- Ask therapists to build flexibility into the HEP. The HEP should constantly provide higher goals, and ask therapists to give you tools and strategies to achieve those goals.

- Repeat these steps as time goes on. Every year or so (more, if it's needed; less, if you continue to make great gains on your own) go back through the cycle of seeing the **physiatrist** and any appropriate therapists so that they can help you tweak your HEP. This will ensure that your at-home work continues to be challenging and fruitful.

The last week or so before ending therapies is way too late to work with therapists to develop a HEP. The HEP should be developed, in a rolling manner, from the beginning of your relationship with therapists. These professionals are trained to develop plans toward recovery. Much of their education is dedicated to the development of these sorts of plans. Many therapists end sessions because they are forced to, by pressure from managed care (insurance companies). Most will be happy that you want to continue to make progress once your relationship with them ends. But unless you prod and prompt therapists, and provide adequate time toward this goal, they will take the traditional perspective and wait until the last few days to "Hand 'Em Photocopies."

The best way to plan for a fruitful "rest of your life" after discharge is to make it clear to the occupational, physical, and speech therapists that you take your recovery very seriously, and you know that recovery will continue long after you've forgotten their names.

What Precautions Should Be Taken?

Much of the HEP will be implemented when the therapist is no longer around. This may add to the therapist's reluctance to develop a HEP beyond what you've done in his or her care; the therapist doesn't want to plan anything new that may put you into danger. Agree with him or her prior to the development of the HEP that you will take any safety precautions seriously, and you will inform your doctor as you progress. Any time you significantly alter your exercise or therapy routine, inform your doctor. The doctor will agree and encourage your ongoing efforts 99 percent of the time, but let the doctor make the final decision about the safety of the program.

As elements are added to the HEP, be sensitive to changes inherent in your body and mind. If you feel that something is hurting you or is too strenuous, stop. Generally, pain can be trusted as a warning of something harmful.

SPACE TO RECOVER—THE HOME GYM

Clearly, it's easier to study at the library, do paperwork at your desk, and cook in the kitchen. Every stroke survivor also needs a space within his or her home dedicated to recovery. It should be a space where you can focus on recovering from your stroke. Like a library, it should only have the distractions you want; like a desk, it should be organized; like a kitchen, it should have all the recovery tools you need.

Some stroke survivors prefer to pursue at least some of their recovery effort in a community gym. Even if one joins a community gym (see the section Space to Focus—The Community Gym, later in this chapter), there are great reasons for having a home gym as well.

How Is It Done?

Your home gym can be a basement, an extra bedroom, or a corner of a room. It does not have to be big and does not have to have any more equipment than you need. It should have what is necessary to facilitate recovery. This may include exercise equipment, a TV, a stereo, a mirror, and inspirational art. Build your gym as a place of sanctuary and a place of work. Ideas for equipment include:

- A treadmill
- A recumbent cycle
- An upper body ergometer (hand cycle)
- An exercise mat
- Parallel bars or other equipment used to maintain balance
- Weights
- Resistance bands
- Electrical stimulation devices
- Balls, decks of cards, or other "toys"

This list can be as long or as short as it needs to be. A small amount of simple equipment that is well thought out and well used is better than a lot of expensive equipment left in a corner. Doctors and therapists can help compile a list of needed equipment.

What Precautions Should Be Taken?

Be prudent when assembling the gym and think safety first. Any exercise or therapy equipment has inherent dangers. For instance, a treadmill provides a moving surface that may be inappropriate for some stroke survivors. Even something as simple as a ball can facilitate a loss of balance that can cause a fall. Consider installing grab-bars for any balance exercises you do. Make sure the floor is nonslip given the footwear you expect to use. Doctors will tell you if an exercise or therapy is safe, and therapists will explain how to do the exercise or therapy in the most effective way possible.

SPACE TO FOCUS—THE COMMUNITY GYM

A community gym is a great place to focus on recovery. A well-equipped gym, with a supportive staff, provides the environment needed to build muscle, stamina, and flexibility. Gyms often have a pool. Pools provide the buoyancy and resistance of water to aid in recovery. Treadmills, weights, exercise balls, saunas, even giant mirrors, which provide valuable visual feedback, are usually available at the local gym. Gyms are motivating because motivated people go to them. Just being around other folks trying to reach their goals can be motivating.

Gyms in your community are not equipped the same as a home gym. Your home gym will have equipment that is specific to your recovery. For instance, your home gym might have an **e-stim** machine, a pegboard, or a deck of cards—all essential to your recovery, but not available at any gym. The role that the community gym plays in your recovery is different from the role of your home gym. The community gym will be a place of "the big three" of exercise:

1. Cardiovascular training

2. Weight training

3. Stretching

(You might also do any or all of these at home, as well.)

These types of exercises are essential aspects of recovery in order to "bank" the energy needed for every other part of the recovery effort.

Some stroke survivors actually get in better shape *after* their stroke than they were before their stroke. This may happen for several reasons, including:

- A new emphasis on staying in shape

- A new emphasis on diet

- More exercise

- More time available to exercise

For some stroke survivors, the gym experience is a central part of life after stroke. Gyms can be centers of social contact and relaxation, and exciting places if you are motivated. They can also help you focus if you are less than motivated. Gyms provide a great combination of assets to help on the road to recovery.

How Is It Done?

A gym that is appropriate for recovery from stroke will have:

- Appropriate gear

- Surroundings in which the stroke survivor feels comfortable and relaxed

- A knowledgeable and supportive staff

Personnel at gyms do not often have expertise about, or experience with, folks with disabilities. Differences in credentialing add to the confusion. You should know that:

- Athletic trainers have a bachelor's degree in athletic training and are certified by the state in which they practice.

- Personal trainers need no education and no certification.

There are many stories of stroke survivors receiving the wrong advice from well-meaning gym employees. Have a physical and/or occupational therapist direct the rehab program. They don't have to go to the gym with you. The physical and/or occupational therapist simply needs to know what equipment is available so they can set up a safe and effective program. Of course, it would be highly beneficial if the therapist could go to the gym to direct the first session!

Try to find a gym that is close to where you live, and try to incorporate as much of the trip to the gym as possible into your lifestyle. That is, if you can find a gym that you can walk to, use the walking as part of your recovery. If you don't have a gym that close, at least make it convenient to your home or place of work.

Finding a gym whose members reflect your age group and gender will help you feel comfortable. Before joining a gym, tour the facility during the time that you would usually go. This will help determine the makeup of the membership and will help determine how crowded it might be during the time that you would typically go. Try to find a gym that offers classes that may facilitate stroke recovery. While spinning or rock climbing may not be within your interest and capacity, yoga, Tai Chi, or water aerobics may fit your ability and goals. Accessibility may be an issue as well. It is the law (within the Americans with Disabilities Act or ADA) that businesses must provide wheelchair-accessible entrances, exits, and bathrooms. This may not be the case, however. Most gyms make the effort to comply. But some of the equipment may not be accessible for folks with an inability to walk or transfer (i.e., get on/off equipment). For instance, a hydraulic lift chair is can safely transfer folks with mobility problems in and out of a pool. But many pools do not have one, so consider this when choosing a gym.

Your insurance may be willing to pay for some or all of your gym membership. In the United States, there is a way to get a free membership to thousands of exercise facilities across the country. It's called SilverSneakers. Typically you have to be 65 or over to qualify, but if you've had a stroke and have disability benefits, you also may qualify. Find out more at silversneakers.com.

What Precautions Should Be Taken?

Inform your doctor before starting or changing any exercise program.

WEIGHT UP!

Resistance training is the general term for any exercise in which muscles work against resistance. The most common type of resistance training is weight training (sometimes called weight lifting). Resistance training provides many important benefits to a poststroke therapy routine. Taken in total, these benefits make resistance training essential in any serious efforts toward recovery from stroke.

Resistance training and weight training are sometimes used inter-changeably. For clarification, here are the distinctions:

- *Resistance training*: Resistance training is pushing (or pulling) against an opposing force. This includes your own resistance (e.g., push-ing one hand against the other), someone else's resistance, gravity, resistance bands (made from sheets of rubber or rubber tubing), and so on.

- *Weight training*: Weight training is resistance training where the force against which you are pushing (or pulling) is weights, which include barbells, dumbbells, and weight machines (like those found in a gym).

This chapter uses the more catch-all term, *resistance training*. Here is a list of reasons to add this sort of training to your daily routine:

Resistance training:

- Increases strength on the "good" and "bad" sides
- Improves mobility (walking, wheelchair movement, etc.)
- Reverses muscle atrophy (muscles getting smaller and weaker). Atrophy affects both the affected and unaffected sides after stroke.
- Increases functional ability. ("Functional" is a buzz word used by healthcare workers that describes the ability to do normal, everyday activities, also known as ADLs or activities of daily living.)
- Increases strength, which helps all other efforts toward recovery
- Boosts chemicals (most importantly, **BDNF**) in the brain that can facili-tate the neuroplastic change needed to learn and relearn movement
- Increases balance and decreases falls
- Increases cogitative function; its good for the brain

Bone density is an important benefit of weight training because the denser the bone, the stronger it is. There is a process that happens in bones called **Wolf's law**. Wolf's law says that a bone will get thicker and stronger because of the stresses that are put on it. As muscle pulls on bone, the bone responds by getting thicker and stronger. Over time, the more stress on the bone by the muscles, the greater the bone growth. Resistance training increases stress on bones, which increases bone density.

Wolf's law works in the opposite way, as well. The less stress that is put on bones, the weaker bones get. After stroke, the muscles on the weak side contract (tighten) less. Thus, the muscles on the affected side put less stress on bones. This lack of stress results in a decrease in bone strength. Because survivors tend to fall toward the "bad" side (the side that has weaker bones), they are at a much greater risk of fracture. Increasing bone strength on the "bad" side with resistance training reduces the chance of fracture.

There are other benefits to resistance training that are not specific to stroke survivors but are important to everyone's health. Resistance training:

- Helps to balance blood sugar, which is important for diabetics and pre-diabetics.*

- Increases resting metabolism, which reduces weight or reduces the speed at which weight is gained.*

- Reduces blood pressure.*

How Is It Done?

Resistance training helps with so many of the body's systems that it is good for everyone. But for folks who have had a stroke, resistance training is doubly important. Incorporate resistance training into a stroke-recovery strategy and be prepared for increases in energy, muscle strength, and endurance.

When deciding where resistance training fits into your recovery plan, carefully consider what area of the body to focus on. The recovery plan should include resistance training for all four limbs as well as your trunk (the area from mid-chest to hips, including the back). But some muscle groups will receive more focus than others. For instance, if it has been determined that the ability to walk will benefit from resistance training of the muscles of the thigh, then that's where more time and resistance training should be put. Accurately evaluating which muscles need work is the first step in developing your resistance training program. Therapists can help you determine which muscles need the most work. You can also help determine what muscles to work on using common sense and intuition. Generally speaking, stroke survivors have much less weakness in the flexor

---

* Diabetes, obesity, and high blood pressure increase the risk of having a stroke.

muscles than the extensor muscles. Flexor muscles are muscles that decrease joint angles. For instance, in the elbow, the flexor muscles bend the elbow. The extensor muscles straighten the elbow. The elbow well exemplifies the problem that stroke survivors typically have: They can bend the elbow pretty well, but cannot straighten the elbow. This is a case where resistance training would be better directed toward the extensor muscles than the flexors muscles. Focus on muscle groups (groups of muscles that work together) that are weakest. See the section Challenge Equals Recovery in Chapter 2, for strategies to focus on what is hardest. This is not to say that the stronger of the two muscle groups, the flexors, should not be worked, as well. Despite the fact that the flexor muscles tend to overpower, both sets of muscles are weak after stroke. However, resistance training should be directed primarily toward the extensor muscles, which tends to be the weaker after stroke.

It is not necessary to buy expensive equipment to add resistance training to your recovery effort. The following work just as well as expensive weights or weight machines:

- Elastic bands or cords
- The force of your own body against itself (isometric exercise, e.g., grasping the fingers of one hand with the other hand and pulling both hands away from each other)
- The force of gravity (e.g., squats, heel-ups, press-ups)

When deciding how to incorporate resistance training into a recovery plan, keep in mind the following:

- Consult your doctor and therapist. They will help you determine the exercises that should be done, the progression of those exercises, and the equipment needed.
- Proper progression of exercises, to keep muscles challenged while maintaining safety, is an essential part of resistance training. Progression of resistance training should involve, over an arc of time, an increase in the number of repetitions, an increase of resistance (weight), or both.

What Precautions Should Be Taken?

Start resistance training slowly and allow for a gradual progression. There is a phenomenon called "delayed-onset muscle soreness," commonly known as DOMS. When DOMS does occur, muscular soreness is felt from a day to a few days after the resistance training. This is a good reason to start slowly and frequently evaluate how your muscles feel. Building muscle involves developing small tears in muscle fibers, so a small amount of muscular pain is to be expected. The muscle is "repaired" by coming back thicker and stronger.

Consult your doctor regarding any health risks that may occur because of resistance training. Your doctor will tell you how the medications you are taking may affect your body's response to exercise. Have your occupational or physical therapist help you design a resistance training program that is safe, has built-in increases of challenges over time, and is appropriate to your particular deficits and personal goals. Take your blood pressure and pulse rate before, during, and after resistance training (see the section Five Tests You Should Do in Chapter 3). Some doctors may not want resistance training incorporated if the stroke survivor has had a hemorrhagic stroke (bleeding stroke), because of the risk of another stroke due to possible spikes in blood pressure during resistance training.

BANK ENERGY AND WATCH YOUR INVESTMENT GROW

Cardiovascular (or cardiorespiratory) fitness refers to the ability of the heart, lungs, and blood vessels to supply oxygen to muscles during exercise. Stroke survivors face unique challenges when it comes to their cardiovascular fitness.

- Stroke survivors have *half* the amount of stamina as people who have not had a stroke and are . . .
  — Age-matched
  — Out-of-shape
  — "Couch potatoes" (people who do not exercise)
- It takes stroke survivors *twice* the amount of energy to do daily activities (walking, dressing, eating, etc.).

In other words, stroke survivors have half the energy to do twice the work. So, there is less energy available and more energy needed. This is why cardiovascular exercises and weight training—muscle building—are so important. There is a reason why athletes start their season with physically demanding workouts. They are banking energy for the game itself. You should do the same. Basic forms of exercise provide the stamina that's needed to pursue the other challenges of recovery.

Exercise helps recovery in many other ways. In fact, exercise helps the brain rewire after stroke. Exercise helps get oxygen-rich blood to the brain, and the brain loves oxygen. The brain is 2 percent of total body weight, but consumes 20 percent of the total oxygen used by the body. Exercise increases blood circulation to your brain. The improved oxygen flow to the brain helps every kind of learning, including the relearning of movement after stroke. Exercise also increases the blood levels of **BDNF**. BDNF, explained in more detail in Neuroscience: Your New Best Friend in Chapter 1, has been called "miracle grow for the brain" because it makes learning (including learning to move after stroke) much easier. Exercise, both cardiovascular and resistance training, increases your access to BDNF. You can bank energy by following a challenging and safe cardiovascular exercise program. *The strength of the heart, lungs, blood vessels, and muscles is the foundation on which every other effort toward recovery is built.* It's that simple. Strength of conviction and inner strength can be sky high, but if you don't have energy, you are stopped before you begin. On the other hand, if you are willing to commit to being in shape, you are a long way on the path toward recovery. With energy in the bank, the sky is the limit.

How Is It Done?

Options for cardiovascular workouts are available for every level of ability and disability. From bed-bound exercises to high-level aerobic workouts, there are many options to work the heart and lungs, no matter what the level of recovery. Your physical or occupational therapist or athletic trainer can suggest machines and exercises that build stamina, allow for maximum gains, and keep you safe. Many of the machines that are used for cardio conditioning, include:

- Recumbent (reclining) bilateral trainers (see the discussion of cardiovascular machines in Chapter 9: Recovery Machines)
- Recumbent stationary bicycles
- Upper body exercisers

There are even treadmills for wheelchairs that build cardiovascular strength. Many of the options are low cost. For instance, portable stationary cycles for the lower and upper extremity are available at nominal cost. A company called Isokinetic has five models of pedal exercisers that are appropriate for arm or leg exercise. The cost is between $20 and $70 (www.isokineticsinc.com/category/pedal_exercisers).

Many local hospitals and rehabilitation hospitals have "cardio gyms" for folks rehabilitating from a variety of conditions. These gyms are open to stroke survivors and are staffed with knowledgeable therapists who can help direct workouts. These gyms typically require a doctor's prescription. Insurance companies are sometimes willing to pay for memberships to these gyms if your workouts are seen as necessary for recovery and/or overall health.

For stroke survivors who cannot yet walk, **partial weight supported walking (PWSW)** equipment can be used at home. For example, both the NeuroGym® Bungee Walker and the Biodex Unweighing System are available for home use (see Chapter 9: Recovery Machines).

What Precautions Should Be Taken?

Ask your physical or occupational therapist to review the many options available to develop cardiovascular strength. Many of these options can be used within your home. Involving your doctor and rehabilitation professional to guide you toward safe and effective cardiovascular strengthening options is essential.

6 Recovery Strategies

THE FOUR PHASES OF STROKE RECOVERY—AND WHAT TO DO DURING EACH

There are four phases after stroke:

- Hyperacute → Acute → Subacute → Chronic

There are two ways of describing the four phases.

1. The "one size fits all" timeline.
2. The "unique" timeline. This timeline reflects the recovery of individual survivors.

Both definitions are useful.

The "One Size Fits All" Timeline

This timeline is an average of the stroke recovery process. It provides a generalized perspective on where the survivor is in recovery. If a survivor says, "My stroke was seven months ago" doctors and therapists can make certain assumptions about where the survivor is in recovery. The "one size fits all" timeline is also useful in research. It can be used to define a group of survivors on which a treatment is used. For instance, the research may involve "survivors that are three to five months post (after) stroke."

The four stages of stroke according to the one-size-fits-all timeline:

1. Hyperacute: From the first symptom to the first six hours
2. Acute: The first seven days

3. Subacute: The first seven days to three months

4. Chronic: From the first three months to the end of life

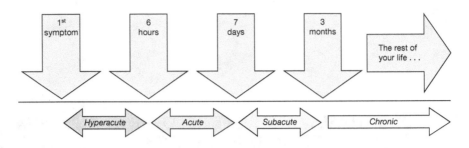

The phases of stroke recovery as a "one-size-fits-all" timeline.

The "Unique" Timeline

The "unique" timeline comes from studies of brain scans of stroke survivors. These studies reveal that the course of every stroke is different. Every stroke survivor enters and exits the phases of recovery at different times.

Choosing the best available strategy option partially depends on where the survivor is in recovery. Different strategies work during different phases. Also, certain treatment options can be detrimental during certain phases, so it's important to know what phase the survivor is in.

Determining the phase a survivor is in is often a matter of simple observation. The way the body moves provides insight into what is going on in the brain. The survivor and everyone around the survivor can help determine which phase the survivor is in.

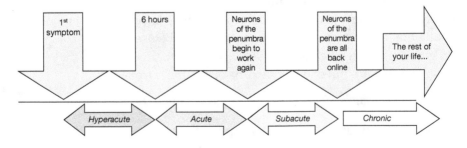

The phases of stroke recovery as a unique timeline.

Hyperacute Phase

BEGINS	ENDS
The first symptom of stroke	Six hours after the first symptom

In both forms of the timeline, the hyperacute stage is the same:

- From the first symptom to six hours after the first symptom

Once the first symptom is recognized, the clock is ticking! Some survivors do not receive emergency care during the hyperacute period. This is unfortunate because this the *only* period in which an aggressive "clot-busting" drug can be given. This drug, called tPA (tissue plasminogen activator), is a *thrombolytic* (*thrombo*: clot; *lytic*: breaking down). (Note: This does not apply to hemorrhagic "bleed" strokes. tPA is contraindicated in bleed strokes.) The recovery for survivors who receive tPA is usually both better and faster. This is why recognizing a stroke, and getting to emergency services, is vital. The faster the survivor can receive emergency care, the better chance they have of getting tPA. Receiving tPA can even happen before you get to the hospital. There are now "mobile stroke units." These ambulances have equipment and personnel that can diagnose and treat with tPA before the survivor reaches the hospital. Literally: *Time Is Brain*. This phase is also critical to providing other medical interventions that can save the brain. Getting immediate care is not only essential to saving as much brain as possible, it is often essential to saving the survivor's life.

What Is the Best Recovery Strategy During the Hyperacute Phase?

The most important thing a survivor and caregivers can do to aid recovery is to seek emergency medical care as soon as possible. Call 911. Time lost is brain lost. There is no rehabilitation during this period. If the patient is conscious, there may be tests of movement by medical staff. These tests provide information about the amount of damage that the stroke is causing over time. However, the focus of this stage is:

1. Saving the patient's life
2. Saving as much brain as possible

Acute Phase

BEGINS	ENDS
The sixth hour after stroke	1. When the blood supply has been restored 2. There is no further damage is caused by the stroke 3. The survivor is "medically stable" 4. The first neurons of the penumbra begin to come back on line

During the acute phase, two distinct areas emerge in the brain: the core and the penumbra.

1. *The core . . .*

- Was killed by the stroke

- Has all its neurons (nerve cells) die

- Has no chance of brain rewiring (neuroplasticity)

- Forms a cavity in the brain that fills with fluid

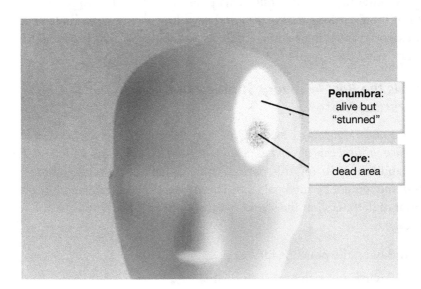

Penumbra: alive but "stunned"

Core: dead area

2. During the acute phase, *the penumbra*:

- Is much larger than the core (the area killed by the stroke)
- Represents billions and billions of neurons
- Is alive, but just barely
- Will end up being useful, or useless, depending on what is done during rehabilitation

The stroke causes interruption of blood supply to the core and penumbra. The blood supply is interrupted because the blood vessels are either blocked (in a "block" stroke) or bursts (in a bleed stroke).

The interruption of the blood supply causes the *core* to die. The *penumbra* stays alive, but just barely. Because the main blood vessel is (at least temporarily) not working, the penumbra relies on smaller blood vessels to stay alive. The neurons in the penumbra get enough blood to stay alive during the acute phase. But those neurons get less blood than they need. Because of the diminished blood supply, the neurons in the penumbra are not able to do their job.

But there is another problem for the billions of neurons in the penumbra.

An injury to any part of the body will cause many body systems to come to the aid of the injured area. Think of the swelling caused by a twisted ankle or a bruised arm. The same happens to the penumbra after stroke. During the early phases after stroke there is swelling in the area. This is caused by many chemicals dispensed in the penumbra. Calcium, destructive enzymes, free radicals, nitric oxide, and other chemicals are delivered to the area. The area is awash in a "metabolic soup" designed to aid healing, but that causes swelling. While the mix of chemicals aids in healing, it provides a poor environment for neurons to work.

So the penumbra is dealing with two issues caused by the stroke:

1. Lack of adequate blood supply
2. A mix of chemicals that interfere with neuron function

These two factors leave a large swath of the brain (the penumbra) unable to operate. Neurons in this area are alive, but they are "stunned." The technical term that is used is "cortical shock" or "cerebral shock." This leaves many survivors with paralysis. But paralysis during the acute phase is not necessarily permanent. For some survivors, the neurons of the penumbra *do* start working again. Recovery of the penumbra happens in the next phase; the subacute phase.

What Is the Recovery Strategy During the Acute Phase?

Intensive therapy is a bad idea during the acute phase.

The brain remains in a very delicate state during the acute phase. The neurons of penumbra are especially vulnerable. Consider the studies of animals that have been given a stroke. Animals forced to do too much too soon *increase* the damage to their brains. In human studies, the results of intensive rehab (too much, too soon) have been mixed at best. Science will continue to add clarity to the question, "How much is too much during the acute phase?" Until then, the rules are simple:

- Follow doctors' orders
- Listen to the therapists and nurses
- Don't push it

Intensive efforts to recover during the acute phase will hurt recovery. But that does not mean that there is *no* therapy. Doctors place many survivors on bed rest for the first two to three days after stroke. However, even during bed rest, therapy will begin. Therapists will often do passive (without any patient effort) movements of the survivor. The survivor's limbs will be moved through their range of motion. These movements, called "passive ranging," will help retain muscle length and keep joints healthy.

Once the doctor gives the okay to come off bed rest, therapists will use their clinical judgment to gently and safely get the survivor moving. During the acute phase, most therapy is done "bedside" (in the patient's room). Therapists will gently get the survivor moving. Therapists who work with acute survivors often sum up their treatment philosophy with a simple phrase: "We do whatever the patient can do safely."

Before providing therapy in the acute phase, therapists will test . . .

- Judgment and safety awareness
- The ability to follow commands
- Orientation (i.e., "Where are you? Who am I? What is the time of day, season, etc.? Many patients may feel insulted by the simplicity of these

questions. These questions are, however, essential to establishing safety.)

- Memory
- Problem solving
- Vision
- Ability to actively move the limbs (active range of motion, or AROM)
- Strength
- Fine motor coordination
- Sensation

Once evaluated, therapy starts with very simple movements and activities. For instance, if it is safe, therapists will help survivors . . .

- Reach, touch, or grasp objects with the "bad" side arm/hand
- Sit on the edge of the bed
- Go from sitting to standing
- Walk

During the acute phase, listen closely to therapists. Therapists as well as doctors and nurses will provide guidance about what recovery strategies should be done. Caregivers can also help by doing therapists-suggested activities during the time when the survivor is the most alert. Activities might include anything from having a conversation with the survivor to encouraging basic movements (e.g., opening and closing the hand).

There is another way caregivers can be vital to recovery during the acute phase. Because they are often with the survivor many hours a day, caregivers can alert therapists to changes in the ability to move. For instance, let's say the survivor cannot bend his or her elbow at all on Monday. Then—without any practice at all—on Wednesday, they can bend the elbow a few degrees. This is known as **spontaneous recovery**. Spontaneous recovery is vital to recognize for two reasons:

1. It is the harkening of the subacute phase (discussed next)
2. It is the harkening of when really hard and productive work can begin

If the caregiver observes spontaneous recovery, report it to the therapist! The most important phase of recovery (subacute phase) has begun!

Subacute Phase

BEGINS	ENDS
The first neurons of the penumbra come "on line"	All the neurons in the penumbra are "on line"

The subacute phase is a time of great hope for many stroke survivors. There is a huge influx of neurons that allow the survivor to recover at a rapid pace. Much of the recovery is considered **spontaneous recovery** (lots of recovery with little effort). The reason for this rapid spontaneous recovery is that neurons that were "off line" are coming back "on line." Some survivors make a near full recovery during the subacute phase. Other survivors are not so lucky. They take longer to reengage the neurons of the penumbra. For these survivors there is a problem with the penumbra.

The Problem With the Penumbra

The brain is very "use it or lose it." If the neurons of the penumbra are not challenged to work again, they stop working. This process (unused neurons losing function) is known as **learned nonuse**. (For a full explanation of learned nonuse, please see the section Constraint-Induced Therapy for the Arm and Hand in Chapter 4.)

But why would the neurons of the penumbra *not* be used? Certainly the survivor will be encouraged to move. And that movement will reengage neurons, right? For the minority of survivors this is exactly true. For these "lucky" survivors, **functional** (usable, "real world") movement is quickly gained, and learned nonuse never takes place.

For many survivors learned nonuse is, well, *learned*. Much of the reason learned nonuse takes root is the *"meet 'em, greet 'em, treat 'em, and street 'em"* mentality forced on therapists by managed care. Therapists are sensitive to Rule No. 1: *Get them safe, functional, and out the door*. Being functional *is* the end goal. But for survivors who don't yet have function, there is only one way to "get out the door": *Compensation* (using only the "good side" limbs to get things done). Using the "good" side to do everything means neurons in the penumbra lack the challenge needed to come back "on line." As the neurons of the penumbra become useable, nothing is asked of them, and learned nonuse sets in.

What Is the Best Recovery Strategy During the Subacute Phase?

The subacute phase is the most important phase in the process of recovery. The intensity and quality of effort during the subacute phase will help determine the amount of recovery. A successful subacute phase ensures the highest level of recovery.

During the subacute phase, the billions of neurons that have survived the stroke become available to go back to work. The point at which each and every neuron is available is the beginning of the chronic phase (discussed next).

Much of recovery during the subacute phase comes from neurons that were "off line" coming "online." This is the essence of spontaneous recovery: Neurons that were not available for work become, during subacute phase, available for work. During the subacute phase, many survivors have an opportunity to "ride the wave of spontaneous recovery." Everyone is willing to take credit for the recovery. The survivor may say something like, "I'm getting a lot of recovery because I'm working really hard," and the therapist may think that the survivor is recovering because of the great therapy. But much of the recovery during the subacute phase is because billions and billions of neurons are rushing back to become usable again. Just as is true when swelling goes down after you injure a muscle, as the swelling goes down after stroke, neurons become available to go back to work.

Because rehab during the subacute phase is so important, it gets its own section! Please see section titled The Subacute Phase: Recovery's Sweet Spot (later in this chapter) for suggestions on how to use the subacute period to achieve the highest possible level of recovery.

Chronic Phase

BEGINS	ENDS
All the neurons in the penumbra are "on line"	The end of the survivor's life

At some point, all the neurons of the penumbra are back online, so there is no "wave" to ride. This is the harkening of the chronic phase.

As the subacute phase ends and the chronic phase begins, the survivor is left with two kinds of neurons. Let's call them "working neurons" and "lazy neurons."

Working Neurons

Some neurons do just fine and go right back (during the subacute phase) to what they were doing before the stroke.

For instance, neurons might go back to . . .

- Straightening the elbow
- Lifting the foot during walking
- Controlling the mouth during speech
- Opening the hand
- And so on

Working neurons resume their pre-stroke responsibilities. These are the neurons that, as they rush back on line during the subacute phase, propel **spontaneous recovery**.

"Lazy" Neurons

These neurons are never asked to do anything after the stroke. Through the process known as **learned nonuse**, they "lie fallow." This is usually the case when, during the subacute phase, the survivor is taught to compensate with the "good" side to become "functional." But there is a downside to this rush toward functional. As is true with the rest of the brain, each and every neuron is "use it or *lose* it." What "lazy" neurons *lose* are connections between themselves and other neurons. These connections are called "synaptic connections."

Normally, neurons use connections to communicate with other neurons. Because those connections are used, they remain working. When a neuron does not communicate with other neurons, connections are lost. This is the essence of the "use it or lose it" aspect of the brain. What is lost are connections between neurons, but not just the connections are lost. Within each of these nonworking neurons is a loss of dendrites. Dendrites are the *branching* arms that provide the connections between neurons. And "branch" is the perfect word. In fact, the technical term used for the shortening of these branches is *pruning*—just like pruning the branches of a bush or tree. The phrases scientists use are "pruning of the dendritic arbor" or, simply, "dendritic pruning." This is what happens to "lazy" neurons affected by learned nonuse. They prune connections.

Losing More Than What the Stroke Took

Learned nonuse expands the influence of the stroke to beyond what is killed by the stroke. Learned nonuse drags the penumbra down with it, radically increasing the effects of the stroke. And that would be bad enough. But it gets worse. The brain also has to deal with **diaschisis**.

Diaschisis: Expanding the Stroke Footprint

Meet Dave, an avid tennis player. Dave had a stroke. For a while after the stroke, Dave is unable to attempt to play tennis.

Dave has not only lost his ability to play tennis. Many other tennis-related skills are also lost because Dave is no longer playing tennis. All the functions the brain has to do to play tennis are lost as well. For example, tennis players have to—very rapidly—process a lot of visual information. Included are speed and spin of the ball, the momentum of the opposing player, racket angle, court lines, the net, and so on. Tennis involves *a lot* of visual processing by the brain. Again, because of the stroke, Dave is not playing tennis anymore. You can guess what happens to the vision area of Dave's brain; it too goes through a "pruning of the dendritic arbor." This process is known as **diaschisis**.

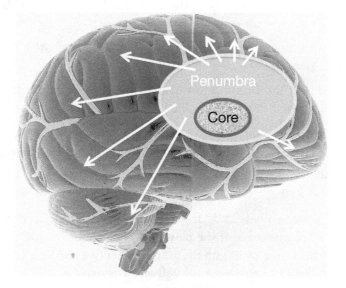

Not only does the core die, but through learned nonuse the penumbra and many other parts of the brain **(diaschisis)** suffer as well.

The cascade of learned nonuse looks like this:

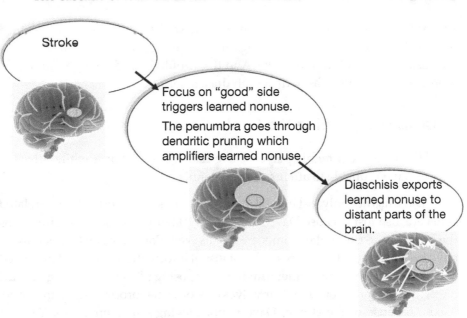

Simply:

- *Stroke*: The survivor has a stroke. A small portion of the brain (core) dies and is forever gone.

- *Learned nonuse*: The penumbra that surrounds the core is not used and lies fallow for the rest of the survivor's life.

- *Diaschisis*: The negative effect of the stroke and learned nonuse is exported to distant parts of the brain

As you can see, the key to recovery is to not drag the entire brain down with the stroke. The best strategy to keep as much brain as possible is to not let learned nonuse be ... learned. And the best way to do this is to engage the penumbra as it comes back "on line" (during the subacute phase).

As the subacute phase ends, the chronic phase begins. The chronic period starts when all the neurons of the penumbra are either "working" or "lazy." At this point, the survivor has no more **spontaneous recovery**. Therapists recognize this point in recovery—it's relatively easy to see. The survivor is no longer recovering. Clinicians call this a **plateau**. Because of the pressures of managed care (insurance), therapists are required to discharge (end therapy with) survivors who have plateaued. The thinking is "This patient is not making any progress. Why are we paying for more therapy?"

For many stroke survivors, the plateau may not be permanent. Researchers have found two specific ways of breaking through a plateau during the chronic phase.

1. Getting the lazy neurons to work again
2. Recruiting other neurons in the brain to take over what is lost during the stroke.

Getting Lazy Neurons to Work Again

Reactivating lazy neurons is known as "reversing learned nonuse." The idea is to challenge the lazy neurons so that they are *forced* to grow new connections to neighboring neurons—"forced" is the operative word here. In fact, one of the ways to force neurons to develop connections is called "**forced use**." Forced use is a part of **constraint-induced therapy** in which the "good" limb is not allowed to do anything. This forces the "bad" limb to do a lot of difficult and uncomfortable work. But difficult and uncomfortable work is how and why the brain rewires. Brain rewiring (also known as *learning*) is difficult, from learning a foreign language to learning how to play the violin. The key to learning, including learning after stroke, is challenge. Challenging "lazy" neurons to reach out to other neurons forms new connections between neurons. Getting "lazy" neurons to build connections is one way the stroke survivor has the potential to recover during the chronic phase.

Recruiting Other Neurons in the Brain to Take Over What Is Lost During the Stroke

The brain is "plastic," and just like plastic you find in everything from car parts to plastic bottles, the brain can change itself physically. For plastic bottles to change form, they need to be heated. For the brain to change it needs challenge. Here is an example of plasticity in play after stroke.

Prior to her stroke, Janice was a florist. Since her stroke she has been unable to move her left hand. Researchers scanned her brain. Sure enough, when she tries to move her left hand, no part of the brain "lights up." But because of her work she is forced again and again to try to use the "bad" hand. Eventually she gets a small but important amount of movement back. Researchers scan her brain again . . . but what lights up is not what you'd expect.

The brain is backward. The left side of the body is controlled by the right side of the brain, and vice versa. When Janice moves her left hand in the brain scanner, the right side of the brain should light up. But it doesn't. What lights up is the left ("wrong") side of her brain. In other words, Janice is "borrowing" neurons from her left hand to move her right hand.

Neurons can be recruited from different parts of the brain to do a task they were never asked to do before. That is the power of plasticity and it is a power that survivors can use well into the chronic phase. Challenge recruits *unrelated neurons in the brain to take over what is lost during the stroke.*

What Is the Best Recovery Strategy During the Chronic Phase?

The following are general rules for recovering during the chronic phase. Note that there are strategies throughout this book that will help survivors make progress during the chronic phase.

- *Recovery requires a do-it-yourself focus.*
  There is a point at which therapists are no longer available to the survivor. Therapists can be helpful at different intervals during the chronic phase (e.g.. every 6 months, every year). Therapists can look at what the survivor is doing and offer suggestions to continue recovery. But therapists are not necessary during the chronic phase. Once therapy has ended, stroke survivors are, and should be, in control of their own recovery. This phase of recovery is based on a lot of self-directed hard work. In order to take charge, stroke survivors need the tools to initiate and follow an "upward spiral of recovery." The "upward spiral of recovery" is driven by real-life demands for everything from coordination to cardiovascular strength. These real-life demands can be aided by the suggestions given throughout this book. From working on muscle strength to incorporating mental practice, there are many recovery options to choose from during the chronic phase.

- *Forget the plateau: It doesn't happen.*
  Plateau means "flattening out." The term is used to describe when it is perceived that a survivor is not making progress. Traditionally, the arc of recovery was believed to have one plateau, at the end of the subacute phase. Research in the last couple of decades has proven that, for some survivors, plateaus can be overcome. During the chronic phase, recovery is made up of multiple plateaus that happen for many years to come. For a full explanation of the plateau and how to bust through it, please see the section Say No to Plateau in Chapter 1.

- *Stay in good shape.*
  Everyone is getting older. As we age, staying in shape is vital to everything, from overall health to allowing us continue to do the activities we love. But survivors have an added energy-burning burden. Basic daily activities (e.g., walking, dressing) take twice as much energy after stroke, and survivors need even more energy because recovery requires effort and effort requires energy. For a full explanation of the importance of and how to maintain heart, lung, and muscle strength after stroke, please see two sections in Chapter 5: Weight Up! and Bank Energy and Watch Your Investment Grow.

- *Don't let soft tissue shorten.*
  If tissue shortening (i.e., muscle tightness) happens, recovery of movement can be compromised and/or entirely halted. You can do a ton of hard work, but if the muscle length is not there, that's as far as you'll go—it's that simple. This is particularly true of the tendency toward the shortening of soft tissue in the elbow, wrist, and finger flexors in the arm and hand. In the leg and foot, the main concern is the calf muscle. Spasticity in the calf keeps the foot pointed down. If held long enough, the calf muscle will shorten. But many other muscles are at risk as well. For a full explanation of the importance of and how to maintain soft tissue (muscle, etc.) length, please see the section Don't Shorten in Chapter 3.

Phase-Focused Recovery

There are three ways that recovery can happen.

Strength is increased: You develop increased muscle strength, and cardiovascular (heart and lung) strength.

- Strengthening should be encouraged during the subacute and chronic phases of stroke.

- Strengthening during the hyperacute and acute phases will hurt recovery.

The penumbra is saved: During the subacute phase the neurons of the penumbra are brought back on line.

The brain is rewired: During the chronic phase brain plasticity allows for a completely new and different area of the brain to take over for lost function.

Here is a "cheat sheet" for phase-focused recovery:

PHASE ↓	FOCUS →	CARDIOVASCULAR AND MUSCULAR ENDURANCE	SAVING THE PENUMBRA	REWIRING THE BRAIN
Subacute		✓	✓	
Chronic		✓		✓

When Does Recovery End?

"How do I know when I'm done recovering?" This is a legitimate question. It's a tough one, too. I asked this question of Kathy Spencer, a friend and one of the most motivated survivors I've ever met. She puts it this way . . .

> I don't think recovery ever ends. I tell stroke survivors that with the plasticity of the brain—we are never done recovering unless we quit working or die. I still work on things, just not as intensely. I think for me, after working over two years every single day, I felt like I needed and wanted to get on with life—and I have SO much recovery that I'm okay with it. I do fine with motor stuff—type, write, piano, etc., but I could benefit if I did more. I just bought one of those hand grip things to carry in my car to strengthen my fingers while driving, but now I can do so much with my fingers. I can even put in pierced earrings, hook my necklaces, jog, jump, etc.—I just don't focus on it nearly as much as I used to. So to answer your question—at what point are the efforts toward recovery no longer worth the time—it's always worth the time, but when you can do so much after not being able to do it for two years—you reach a point of satisfaction but still work—just not as hard! I would never tell a person that working on recovery ends or is a waste of time.

THE SUBACUTE PHASE: RECOVERY'S SWEET SPOT

Terms you will need to know to understand this section . . .

Penumbra: A viable area of the brain next to the area killed by the stroke. The penumbra is much larger than the area killed by the stroke and represents billions of neurons. These are neurons that survive stroke, but their usefulness remains the question. The subacute phase will decide that question.

Neurons: The nerve cells in the brain that allow you to think and move.

Neurons "on line" and "off line":

- On line: Neurons alive and working
- Off line: Neurons alive but not working

Subacute: The point at which the neurons of the penumbra come back on line.

Spontaneous recovery: Recovery that comes with little or no work.

Intensity: The amount of energy, strength, concentration and time put into rehabilitation.

The subacute phase is the most important to recovery after stroke—so much can go right and so much can go wrong.

- What can go right:
  — The neurons that survive the stroke *are used* and so become *useful*.
- What can go wrong:
  — The neurons that survive the stroke *are not* used and so become *useless*.

The area in play is called the **penumbra**. During the subacute phase, neurons of the penumbra can either be used or not used.

- Prior to the stroke, these neurons may have been involved in anything from opening the hand to controlling the muscles of the mouth during speech. Neurons that *are* used (and therefore useful) respond to that use by accepting these pre-stroke responsibilities.

- Neurons that *are not* used lose their connections to other neurons (and are therefore useless). They are still alive, but they are isolated. Neurons work together in large groups to help you move, speak, think, and so on. Neurons that are isolated can do very little to help those tasks.

The penumbra can either be "turned on" or "turned off." The subacute phase is the best time to turn the penumbra on. Turning on the penumbra will help achieve the highest level of possible recovery.

Of all the phases of stroke, the subacute phase involves the hardest work, and the biggest payoff. Think of the subacute phase as recovery's "sweet spot." Taking it easy during this phase will expand the impact of your stroke and will decrease overall recovery. Working hard during the subacute phase is critical to having the brain reach every last bit of its potential.

There are two keys to getting the most from the neurons of the penumbra:

1. Using the neurons of the penumbra
2. Timing the use of the neurons of the penumbra

As the neurons of the penumbra come back on line, using those neurons is key to optimal recovery. The other key is the timing of the use. Neurons of the penumbra stressed into use too *early* (during hyperacute and acute phases) can limit recovery. If stressed into use too *late* (during the chronic phase), the impact on recovery will be limited.

How Is It Done?

Let's say Mr. Smith has had a stroke. He has gone through the acute phase and is medically stable. He, his therapists, and his wife all notice that he seems to be getting movement back every day, and the movements seem to be coming back without much work. This is a clear message: *The neurons of the penumbra are coming back on line.* This sort of recovery (movement coming back with little or no effort) is called **spontaneous recovery**. Spontaneous recovery alerts you that the subacute phase has begun.

When you begin to see spontaneous recovery, it's time to "put the pedal to the metal." The problem is, you may not be considered "subacute" when spontaneous recovery arrives. Every stroke is different, every stroke survivor is different, and every recovery is different, so you may be in "acute care" when you're in the subacute phase. It is important for survivors, caregivers, and healthcare professionals to recognize the signs of spontaneous recovery. Spontaneous recovery indicates the subacute phase, and is an indication that serious efforts toward rehabilitation should begin.

Unfortunately, the subacute phase has a couple of forces working against it:

1. Therapists are under very strict orders by neurologists and physiatrists during the acute phase. Therapists are limited in how much and how intensive therapy can be. And this is a good thing. Too much too soon can hurt recovery; this much seems clear in both human and animal studies.

The problem arises when the survivor is considered "acute" when he or she is actually in the subacute phase. In other words, there are two distinct phases with two contradictory rules:

- Acute: Don't do too much or be too intensive.

- Subacute: Turn up the amount and intensity.

Again, this is why recognizing the subacute phase by recognizing spontaneous recovery is so important; it will alert you to what phase you are *really* in.

2. Therapists are restricted as to the amount of therapy that is paid for by insurance (managed care, Medicare, etc.). This perspective is often referred to as "meet 'em, greet 'em, treat 'em, and street 'em." That is, managed care (insurance) requires that therapists get survivors . . .

- Safe

- Functional

- Out the door

All three (safe, functional, and out the door) are important, of course. But many of the efforts to satisfy "safe, functional, and out the door" involve **compensatory strategies** (or, simply, compensation). Compensation is using the "good" side to "get on with your life." This can lead to **learned nonuse**, which describes what happens in the brain when the undamaged side is used and the damaged is not used. Briefly, the less you move the "bad" side of the body, the less of the damaged side of the brain is used. And the parts of the brain that are not used, much like muscle that is not used, get weaker. With compensation, the undamaged side of the brain gets stronger, and the damaged side of the brain gets weaker. This is the opposite of what you want to have happen. You want the damaged part of the brain to be challenged and grow stronger. But you have less time to work on the damaged side when the emphasis is on getting the undamaged side to do almost everything (compensation). There are not enough hours spent in rehab to work on "function" while also working on recovery. Getting the most out of the subacute phase typically involves more—more focus on the affected side, more intensity, and more hours per day focused on recovery. But there is a bit of good news . . . Much of recovery is done when the therapist is not there. Repetitive practice of the movement that you have, mental practice, engaging in conversations and social interactions (enriching your environment), as well as many other techniques, can be used to aid recovery even when therapists are not around.

This will help the damaged part of the brain grow stronger, which will make movement easier and better.

How do you recognize when spontaneous recovery begins? How much intensity should there be during the subacute phase? Here are some questions and answers to help you understand this critical phase of recovery.

Q: *When does the subacute phase begin?*

A: When there is *spontaneous recovery*.

Q: *What is spontaneous recovery?*

A: Recovery with no work.

Q: *How can you recover with no work?*

A: Neurons of the penumbra rush back and become usable.

Q: *What does spontaneous recovery look like?*

A: Movement and sensation that were not available one day become available the next.

Q: *Can spontaneous recovery be anything other than movement or sensation?*

A: It may be anything from regaining speech to remembering your phone number for the first time in days.

Q: *Provide a specific example of spontaneous recovery of movement.*

A: You can't move your foot at the ankle on Monday, but on Tuesday you can move it up and down noticeably.

Q: *Who is most likely to see spontaneous recovery?*

A: The survivor or a caregiver, but it could be a physical therapist, occupational therapist, speech therapist, a doctor, or a nurse.

Q: *Why do you mention the survivor and caregivers before the health professionals?*

A: Survivors are the most aware about what is going on with their body. Caregivers spend the most time with survivors.

Q: *Who do I tell if I observe spontaneous recovery?*

A: Everyone, but especially therapists.

Q: *Is spontaneous recovery ever too subtle to be observed?*

A: Yes, but if you suspect something is changing, tell the therapists. They have tools to measure even the slightest amount of movement or increase in strength.

Q: *Once I recognize the subacute phase, what should be done?*

A: Ease yourself into more intensive stroke recovery options, and slowly increase the number of hours per day spent on recovery.

Q: *Why is it important to "ease into" more intensity and more time?*

A: There are two reasons: (1) The brain is still somewhat vulnerable during this period. Easing into increases in intensity will help the brain adjust accordingly. (2) Because of the stroke and all the things that come from stroke (more medications, difficulty with movement and communication, etc.), the amount of energy the survivor has to recover is limited. Therefore, it is wise to incrementally increase the amount and intensity of efforts toward recovery. As more energy becomes available, more time can be put into recovery efforts.

Q: *What can stand in the way of the neurons of the penumbra completely coming back on line?*

A: Not enough energy, strength, concentration, and time put into rehabilitation during the subacute phase.

Q: *If time with the therapist is limited, how can I ensure that the neurons of the penumbra are challenged?*

A: Accept that the person in the best position to reengage the penumbra is the person who has ownership of the brain in question: *the survivor*.

Q: *If the responsibility of the penumbra is up to the survivor, what are some specific strategies that will help keep the neurons of the penumbra engaged?*

A: Please see the next section entitled Expanding the Therapeutic Footprint.

What Precautions Should Be Taken?

Hard work is important to capture the potential of the penumbra. But the brain—as well as other body systems—can be vulnerable during this period. Healthcare workers, including doctors, nurses, and therapists, can provide insight into what is safe and what is not.

EXPANDING THE THERAPEUTIC FOOTPRINT

Recovery requires a lot of time. It is unrealistic to think that healthcare workers will be there during all of that time. Consider the entire time recovering as the "arc of recovery." The arc of recovery extends from the first symptom of stroke to the highest level of recovery achieved. During the arc of recovery, you will spend a lot more time without professional guidance than you will with it. Physical and occupational therapists, for instance, will be there a small percentage of the total time it takes to recover. The amount of time spent with therapists will be limited in two ways:

1. When you are in therapy you will see therapists for a few hours a day, at most. (What should you do when the therapist leaves the room?)

2. Therapy typically lasts until the beginning of the chronic phase. (What can be done to recover "for the rest of your life?")

Therapists don't need to be there most of the time. What you do on your own will define the extent of your recovery. Survivors have control over their own nervous system, and that nervous system will respond to their hard work. Therapists can't do it for you. Therapists are coaches; they provide guidance. Such guidance can be used to inform efforts toward self-driven recovery.

How Is It Done?

Question: What can you do when the therapist is not there? *Answer*: A lot. I call this idea "expanding the therapeutic footprint." This is a fancy way of saying "use what therapists suggest, even when they're not around." The concept of recovery is relatively simple. Putting into play relatively simple concepts will go a long way toward helping your overall recovery, and therapists will love it too. Most therapists get into the business because they want to help people recover. The more hard work you put in, the more rewarding the experience for both of you.

Here are some suggestions to expand the therapeutic footprint . . .

Use Electrical Stimulation (e-stim)

For most survivors, e-stim can be an easy "do-it-yourself" tool for recovery. E-stim can be used to:

- Temporarily reduce spasticity and provide a stretch to spastic muscles
- Help regain sensation on the "bad" side
- Maintain muscle size (bulk) by forcing muscles weakened by the stroke to flex
- Reduce the chance of blood clots (deep vein thrombosis—DVT) in the calf muscle

Reduce shoulder dislocation (called **subluxation**). Shoulder muscles can become so weak after stroke that the shoulder joint can no longer hold the weight of the arm. This causes the shoulder to dislocate. (See the section Shocking Subluxation in Chapter 4. Also in Chapter 4 is the section Electrical Stimulation for Frugal Dummies, which provides information about how to use e-stim to help "jumpstart" recovery.)

Physical, occupational, and even speech therapists have been using electrical stimulation (e-stim) for decades. There are many uses for e-stim after stroke, from pain relief to muscle building. But the most important use of e-stim for stroke survivors is this: E-stim changes the brain. Brain-scanning studies have shown that e-stim affects the brain after stroke even before the survivor has any muscle control. E-stim can be used to "re-engage" the brain to begin the process of regaining control of muscles. Because it changes the brain before the survivor has control over muscles, e-stim is a great bridge between no movement and some movement. There's a huge difference between "no movement" and "some movement." Small amounts of movement are vital, giving you a fighting chance to regain even more movement. See how in the next section.

Use "Non-Functional" Movement (NFM)

"Non-functional" movement (NFM) is movement that does not help any real-world task. For instance, if a survivor can open and close his or her hand a little bit, but not enough to pick anything up, that movement is considered NFM. NFM can be movement that is too small, weak, or uncoordinated to do any real-world task. While NFM may not help any task, it is vital to recovery. There is a tendency for both healthcare workers and survivors to assume that NFM is not important. The attitude is, "It does not help you do anything, so why do that movement?" This is a mistake. The brain regains control over muscles when those muscles are moved, but if "non-functional" muscles are never moved, how will the brain ever learn to move them better? This is why, when you are not in therapy, it helps to use any NFM you have.

The movements should be repetitive, and challenging. For instance, let's say you have a small amount of movement toward opening your hand. That small amount of movement can be expanded by repetitively using that movement. Focus on challenge by "nipping at the edges" of your current ability. For instance, if you can open your fingers wide enough to pick up a marble, work on opening them wide enough to pick up a ping pong ball. The "off-line" time that you are not in therapy is the perfect time to work on the difficult task of regaining brain control over muscles. And if you do this work when you are *not* in therapy, it is a win-win-win-win!

- WIN: You save yourself money by not burning through valuable therapy time to do the "grunt work" needed to increase small amounts of movement.

- WIN: Therapists can use the gains you have made on your own to expand the options they can use during actual therapy time.

- WIN: Therapists can use the gains you have made on your own to justify more therapy.

- WIN: You learn recovery from "the inside out." What you learn while you're with the therapists will help you recover once therapists are no longer around.

Make the Home Exercise Program (HEP) Immediate and Ongoing

Most of the time the home exercise program (HEP) is an afterthought. It is usually a series of exercises that is given to the survivor once it is believed that recovery has ended. The HEP can be a very powerful tool for recovery. Here are two problems with the typical HEP and two suggestions to make the HEP a more potent tool for recovery.

Problem 1: The HEP is given at the very end of therapy. It's usually one of the last things that's addressed just before the survivor is discharged (the point at which therapy ends).

Solution: Instead of making the HEP something that's dealt with at the end of therapy, it should be initiated at the beginning of therapy. That is, the survivor would benefit from a structured set of responsibilities even during the early phase after stroke (acute). It may be worthwhile to look at the HEP as something other than simply an "exercise program." It can be a set of suggestions that can benefit recovery, even if the therapist is not in the room. For instance, the HEP may include the suggestions made in this section (using mental practice, reinforcing the importance of sleep, engaging in conversations, etc.).

Problem 2: The HEP *is* usually designed to help the survivor maintain any gains achieved in therapy. The HEP *is not* typically designed to help the survivor achieve new gains.

Solution: In the section entitled Get a Home Exercise Program in Chapter 5 are suggestions for the HEP that will help you to continue to make gains, not simply maintain a plateau. (See Chapter 5 more suggestions for the HEP).

Listen to Music

Survivors that listen to their favorite music do better, in many ways, than those who don't listen to music. The benefits of listening to music after stroke are numerous and include . . .

- Better verbal memory (important for survivors who are aphasic)
- More focused attention (important to every aspect of recovery from stroke)
- Improved mood (50 percent of survivors suffer from depression after stroke)

For the best results, start listening to music within the first ten days after stroke. Listen to music that you choose (your favorite music). In research, survivors listened to music at least one hour per day for two months. Study participants started listening to music between five and eight days after their stroke.

Encourage Sleep

Adequate sleep benefits every aspect of recovery. This has been shown to be true in both human and animal studies. Please see the section entitled Horizontal Rehab: Good Sleep = Good Recovery in Chapter 5 for strategies to promote sleep.

Enrich the Environment (EE)

There are many animal studies that show that an "enriched environment" (EE) benefits all aspects of recovery from stroke. There are also an emerging number of human studies that show the same.

So what makes up an EE? Here's the good news: What is considered an EE tends to be fun. Activities that promote an EE include . . .

- Physical activity
- Emotional stimulation
- Conversations
- Social interaction
- Playing games

What does an EE do for stroke survivor? An EE . . .

- Aids in the recovery of movement
- Improves thinking
- Drives helpful neuroplastic (brain rewiring) in the brain
- Reduces for everyone, including stroke survivors, the natural shrinking of the brain that comes with age

Use Mental Practice (MP)

Movements and skills you're trying to relearn after stroke benefit from practice. The practice you do with therapists and on your own is *actual practice*. You can increase the strength of actual practice with mental practice (MP). MP involves imagining whatever skill you're doing during actual practice. MP, its setup and usage is fully described in the section Imagine It! in Chapter 4.

MP is simple. Imagine doing a skill you're trying to recover the way you did it before the stroke. MP is done on your own, in a quiet environment. It takes no physical energy, and is done without a therapist, so it is a perfect way of expanding the therapeutic footprint.

What Precautions Should Be Taken?

The precautions for expanding the therapeutic footprint are treatment-option specific. That is, the precaution would depend on what it is that you're trying to do. It is always wise to ask the appropriate healthcare professional for guidance. These professionals will not only help you make these techniques safer, but they can provide valuable suggestions in making these techniques stronger.

THERAPY SOUP—MIX AND MATCH

Some things are just better together: wine and cheese, baseball and beer, good friends. One option at a time can work well, but sometimes adding a second (or third, or fourth . . .) option can magnify and complement both. The same is true of recovery options. These recovery options include:

- Treatment techniques
- Interventions
- Modalities
- Therapies
- Exercises
- Technologies used for recovery
- Any other effort made toward recovery

How Is It Done?

Mixing and matching (recovery) options is a little like cooking soup. When you cook soup, you taste as you cook. As you add and subtract things to your recovery mix, "taste" the effectiveness of your mix of options.

Adding new options can keep things exciting and, if done correctly, can amplify the efficiency of your recovery routine. The trick is adding a new element and then accurately evaluating if the new element provides a benefit. Finding the correct mix is part science, part art, part intuition, and part experience. There are no rules or flowcharts to direct you through the process of deciding if, what, and when a set of recovery options works.

Some variables that you need to consider when mixing and matching therapies include:

- *Dosage*: Most people think of dosage as something that relates to drugs, but recovery options have dosages as well. Dosage is simply the "how much" of the option you've chosen. Dosage is defined by:
  - *Amount of time*. This would include the amount of time and the number of times per week you spend doing the option. For instance, if you and your doctor have decided that electrical stimulation helps

reduce your spasticity, then the amount of time that you have the stimulation on would help determine the dosage.

— *Intensity*: Again, using electrical stimulation as the example, the level of stimulation (usually measured in milliamps) would help determine the dosage.

- *Type of stroke*:
  — For example, an option may be safe and effective for someone who had a "block" stroke (ischemic, where the blood vessel was blocked). The same option may not be safe for someone who has had a "bleed" stroke (hemorrhagic, where a blood vessel has burst).

- *Side (left or right side of brain) of damage and if the stroke affected the dominant side*:
  — For example, trying to use **repetitive practice** during writing when it is your nonwriting hand that is affected, would not be helpful to recovery.

- *How long after the stroke it has been*:
  — Some options work well right after the stroke. Other options are best tried once you are in the chronic (several months to one year after stroke) stage of recovery.

- *The amount of spasticity you have*:
  — If spasticity is strong, it is sometimes wise to focus on options that reduce spasticity before starting other options.

- *The type and number of conditions related to the stroke*:
  — For example, eyesight problems, loss of feeling, spasticity, aphasia, and so forth.

- *The type and number of health issues that are unrelated to the stroke*:
  — For example, diabetes, heart problems, depression, and so on.

- *Your motivation level*:
  — Some options take a tremendous amount of focused effort. You may not be willing to make that effort, sometimes for under-standable reasons ("I have grandchildren to take care of; I don't have time!"). Even if an option is something you do not want to consider, that does not mean that your efforts should end. It simply means that different options should be explored.

- *The amount of movement you have*:
  - For instance, options that are effective for someone who has near-perfect movement may not be appropriate for someone who is completely limp on the affected side.

The list of variables continues extensively. There are so many considerations in stroke recovery that it is impossible to develop a perfect system to guide you through the process, and even if there were, new research, technologies, and techniques are developed every day. This makes the situation so fluid that the best advice is to always consider new options and accurately and regularly assess progress.

- *Always include options that challenge you*: No progress comes from simply doing what you can. Recovery comes from continually striving for what you are not yet able to do.
- *Consider technology*: The future of rehabilitation is technology. Why? Because there are 50 million stroke survivors worldwide, and the profit motive is too great for inventors to overlook. Fortunately, this means that inventors spend an enormous amount of money on stroke-recovery research. Keep your eye out for emerging technologies to add to your options.
- *As much as you can, choose options with a direct impact on what you love to do*: The part of your life that you most want to get back is a powerful motivator.
- *Always include aerobic (heart and lung) exercises into your mix of options.*
- *Look for options that do well in clinical research*: See the Resources section for easy ways to find out what researchers reject and support.
- *Emphasize options that you can do safely by yourself, at home.*

What Precautions Should Be Taken?

If you take two or more perfectly safe therapies and add them together, they can become dangerous. For instance, imagine if you decide to follow aqua (pool) therapy during the same arc of time that you are doing treadmill training. The two forms of exercises may work well together, but in the short term, they represent a large increase in the amount of stress on your muscles. If you neglect to take into account the increased fatigue that the aqua therapy adds, these two therapies can be dangerous. For example, imagine getting out of the pool, getting dressed, climbing on the treadmill, and then falling because of fatigued arms and legs.

Keep your doctor informed about changes in your recovery options.

LIFESTYLE AS THERAPY

There are not enough hours in a day to accomplish what you need to do while working the full-time job of recovering from a stroke. However, there are errands, chores, and everyday tasks that can be done in a way that promotes recovery. Sure, daily tasks will take a bit longer, but think of the time and money saved if recovery efforts and everyday chores are combined!

Incorporate recovery efforts into the natural rhythm of your life. For instance, within the boundaries of safety, take the stairs, walk to the store, and use the affected hand to do everything from turning the pages of the newspaper to playing catch with grandchildren. Folding clothes is an excellent way to incorporate **bilateral training** (see the section The Good Trains the Bad— Bilateral Training in Chapter 4). Putting away silverware is a good way to work on **repetitive practice** of grasp and release of the hand. Accomplishing simple tasks while focusing on the affected extremities will help improve overall coordination, skill, strength, and functional ability. It is important to understand how valuable everyday tasks are to your recovery. Research has three buzzword concepts that form the foundation of all recovery:

- *Repetitive*: Doing the movements that you want to relearn over and over
- *Task specific*: Having recovery efforts center on specific, real-world tasks
- *Challenging*: Work on tasks that are challenging—as challenging as you can tolerate within the limits of safety

You can see how using everyday tasks as therapy has the potential to incorporate all three of these concepts.

How Is It Done?

Clearly, the best way to improve walking after stroke is to walk a lot (see the section Walking Your Way to Better Walking in Chapter 8). What if you walk to the store, library, or school? For instance, books have to be returned to the library, which is five blocks away. Certainly it would be faster to take the car, but the walk has inherent therapeutic value. Walking is a great exercise and can be naturally incorporated into your lifestyle.

A task like putting away groceries is a great way to do everything from challenging balance to practicing hand grasp and release. Forgoing the elevator for the stairs challenges you by asking for a large amount of lift at the ankle. Painting helps movements at the wrist, elbow, and shoulder, even if you need to place the brush in your "bad" hand with help from your "good" hand. For someone who loves to paint, painting is an example of a meaningful activity. Research has shown that the more meaningful the activity is to you, the more recovery that activity will promote. Some activities are meaningful to everyone, such as walking, eating, and bathing. Other activities have a special meaning to people with special passions, such as playing a musical instrument, playing golf, or painting.

The trick, of course, is taking the extra time needed to fully incorporate the affected arm and leg into whichever task you choose. Taking extra time for these tasks will also help you stay safe. Rushing will hurt everything from coordination to balance, so take your time for the sake of quality of movement and your own safety.

What Precautions Should Be Taken?

Stroke survivors should challenge themselves with everyday tasks. However, it would be wise to always question the safety of attempting even the simplest of tasks. For instance, even a walk to the end of the block can be dangerous if you fatigue easily or you're prone to falling. Reaching up to put a cup in a cupboard may help activate grasp and release, challenge balance, and improve coordination, but this same task can be dangerous if you lose your balance. Stroke survivors should be aware of the dangers of pushing themselves into new and challenging tasks, including inherent dangers from loss of balance, falls, spikes in blood pressure, and so forth.

YOUR WORK SCHEDULE

Studies have shown that, in hospitals, stroke survivors spend just over an hour per day involved in recovery efforts. In skilled nursing clinics, where many stroke survivors end up after their hospital stay, the situation is not much better. The amount of time paid for by Medicare for all therapies, combined, is just over two hours per day, but in order for the brain to rewire, much more time is needed for recovery of movement. For instance, traditional **constraint-induced therapy**, which is proven to promote recovery, has patients do six to eight hours a day of therapy! Recovery efforts are more effective when they are done many hours a day. The brain rewiring needed to recover can happen during short bursts of time, measured in number of weeks (one to ten weeks), but the number of hours per day should be as high as you can tolerate.

How Is It Done?

You can tell how much time per day to spend on recovery with a simple test: How much time does it take to get really good at any skill you've ever acquired? Many of the skills and abilities that we've acquired throughout our lives take years of dedicated practice, and we are happy to do it because we are acquiring a new skill. Stroke recovery has the disadvantage of not involving any movement or skill that is new. You are simply relearning what you once knew how to do well. Still, the challenge of recovery can be exhilarating, but only if you are willing to put in the work and the time needed to show results.

The optimal amount of time that should be spent on any given treatment, exercise, or modality is one of the hot topics of stroke recovery research. Deciding the exact amount of time to spend on recovery efforts can be tricky. It is, however, safe to say that dedicating enough time to recovery can be summarized with the phrase: *Recovery is a full-time job.*

Of course, doing eight hours of work may sound exhausting. Your recovery plan should include options that mix hard physical work with restful work, like **mental practice** (see Imagine It! in Chapter 4). Always balance between work and rest and between maintaining challenge and safety. Often you will not have to do a particular therapy for a long duration of time, as measured in weeks, months, or years. You might instead have an intense experience with a recovery tool for relatively short bursts (two to three weeks) of time. Of course, if a recovery option works for longer than that, keep doing it. On the other hand, if a therapy loses its effectiveness or does not work in a relatively short amount of time, then pitch it. Worthwhile therapies tend to show pretty immediate results. Results have to be measured to determine effectiveness. For suggestions on measurements, see the section Measuring Progress in Chapter 1.

Many stroke survivors are reluctant to put considerable amounts of time into recovery without the guarantee of gains, and there are no guarantees. You may work very hard and recover very little. Efforts toward recovery are a leap of faith. Much of what we do involves leaps of faith, from raising children to getting an education. A full life is full of leaps of faith. Stroke recovery is another leap. Keeping the faith is essential to recovery.

What Precautions Should Be Taken?

The exact amount of effort toward recovery is a decision to be made by the stroke survivor and his or her doctor. Doctors are experts at determining how much work is safe. A balance should be reached between effectively challenging the stroke survivor without pushing him or her to the point of exhaustion. Overexertion will lead to diminished recovery and, finally, to discouragement and quitting.

LIVING RECOVERY

What do you remember from your childhood? Usually it's one of two types of experiences: something good or something bad. Your first kiss and a broken wrist are examples of memories that come back as crystal clear as a photograph. These experiences tend to "hard-wire" into the brain because of their intensity. They have a deep impact that makes you remember the sights, sounds, and emotions of the experience. Intense memories are actually physical in form. They are the connection of particular brain nerve cells firing in a particular order. Think of rehabilitation in much the same way.

When the act of recovery becomes as intense an experience as possible, recovery from stroke can shift into high gear.

How Is It Done?

The more of the whole person, heart and soul, is committed to the movement, the more that movement will be learned. Intensity of emotion and depth of experience can promote recovery by "hard-wiring" the experience. Doctors on the cutting edge of stroke recovery research talk about patients "driving their nervous system" toward recovery. How can a stroke survivor drive their nervous system, in this case, the nerve cells in the brain, toward recovery?

- The effort should be *essential*, meaningful, and passionate. Think of recovery as a challenging vision quest.

- With each instance of committed effort, the brain is slightly altered toward recovery.

- The effort has to be strong enough, focused enough, and personally powerful enough to drive change.

- Any athlete or musician will tell you the same thing: You have to live it.

- When working toward recovery, effort has to be as intensely experienced as you can make it within the limits of safety.

There are many ways that people use depth of experience to change their lives. The experiences at retreats and camps, for example, can change you in profound ways in relatively short periods of time. Consider these two experiences:

- Joe plays two hours of basketball, every Saturday, for a year. That's a total of 104 hours of playing time.

- Jim goes to basketball camp for two weeks and plays for seven hours a day. That's seven hours a day for 14 days, for 98 hours of total playing time.

So Joe, the "weekend warrior," plays for a total of 104 hours and Jim, the "camper," plays 98 hours. Most researchers now believe that Jim the camper would get better at basketball because he would be much more immersed in the experience than Joe. Jim's camp would make him a better basketball player because of the rich emotional experience, which is, quite literally, imprinted on his brain.

What Precautions Should Be Taken?

Any time one considers any difficult physical endeavor, whether it's running a marathon or dedicating fully to recovery from stroke, the precautions are the same: Keep your practice within safe boundaries. There is an old Clint Eastwood line, "A man's got to know his limitations." This is true for anyone trying to recover from stroke. It's a recurring theme in this book: intense, strong, serious, and, most importantly, safe. Consult your doctor about any effort in your recovery that you are unsure about.

KEEP THE CORE VALUES CLOSE

This book, like any book, can be a reference because it is permanent. Read it, and then put it on the shelf to refer to when you need it. The fundamental recovery principles should be memorized and more than memorized; they should become an intrinsic part of the recovery process. Much of recovery you should "feel in your bones." You already do feel it, although recovery may not seem natural. If you've ever challenged yourself to learn a new skill, you already know the process of recovery. Whether you've had a stroke or not, you have the ability to profoundly change your brain. If you are a survivor, you can use the same drive you had all your life to propel brain change. Survivors will benefit from a particular set of core values as they continue on their neuroplastic journey. Keep this book close by on a shelf. Keep the core values in this book closer.

How Is It Done?

The basic elements of successful recovery from stroke are remarkably simple. Here is a quick core values cheat sheet of stroke rehabilitation:

- Develop a plan.
- Don't accept that there will be no more significant recovery.
- Continually research new recovery alternatives.
- Incorporate tasks that are meaningful to you into your recovery efforts.
- Use affected "bad" extremities as much as possible.
- Exercise is good.
- Strengthen your muscles.
- Strengthen your cardiovascular system.
- Stretch often.
- Control your weight.
- Treat efforts toward recovery like a full-time job.
- If you can, walk a lot.
- Take every precaution not to fall.
- Within the boundaries of safety, always challenge yourself.

- Measure progress often.
- Fall in love with the process of recovery.

What Precautions Should Be Taken?

Common sense and your doctor should be your guides.

HARD BUT SAFE

Efforts toward recovery should extend you beyond your current ability while remaining safe. This balance is not difficult to achieve, but does require some planning and consultation with your doctor and other healthcare providers.

When developing a strategy for recovery from stroke, ask yourself two basic questions:

- Is it safe?
- Is it challenging?

If it is safe but not challenging, it will not produce results. If it is challenging but not safe, there is a risk of injury. Pick recovery options that are physically challenging but have little risk.

How Is It Done?

Some inherently dangerous therapies can be modified to make them safe. An example of this is cardiovascular (heart and lungs) training. You could try to swim, attempt to walk briskly, or ride a bicycle. All of these are healthy for your heart and lungs, but they are all dangerous for some folks who have had a stroke. On the other hand, you can modify any recovery option to be safe. For instance, you can change swimming to aqua therapy (therapy done against the resistance of water), and you can use a stationary recumbent bicycle instead of a regular bicycle. Consider walking. Walking is one of the best, if not the best, cardiovascular workouts. If there is a risk of falls or if you are unable to walk, develop a cardiovascular workout that is done in the sitting position. Suggestions for cardio training in the seated position include "ergometers" (stationary cycles for the arms or legs) and recumbent steppers. See Chapter 9 for further examples of machines that help with a cardiovascular workout and that use the legs but do not involve walking. Once you are able to stand, walking can be done with your weight supported or on a treadmill with bars to hold. The worst thing to do, of course, is to assume that walking safely is a lost cause. Giving up on any skill (like walking) may well guarantee more than just losing that skill. It may also provide an opportunity for a downward spiral. Lowered expectations lead to less activity, which leads to less strength and stamina, which, in turn, lead to even lower expectations. Workouts designed to increase heart and lung stamina as well as strengthen muscles will help build the foundation needed to walk safely again. There are other "preambulation" techniques that can be used to foster walking, like partial weight supported walking, the NeuroGym® Bungee Walker, and the Biodex Unweighing System.

The "hard but safe" idea is a cornerstone of rehabilitation therapy and rehabilitation research:

- *Hard (challenging)*: All recovery comes from challenge. In many ways, all recovery is "forced." You put yourself in situations where you can barely achieve the goal, and the challenge itself drives recovery. *The irony of stroke is that the deficits left by the stroke provide the perfect challenges needed to come back from the stroke.* Stroke survivors and well-meaning clinicians often spend much of their effort trying to eliminate the challenge. The saddest situation is when stroke survivors cannot challenge themselves because they don't understand the importance of the challenge. In other cases, survivors are so flaccid (limp) on the affected side that they can't even begin to attempt to meet the challenge. Sometimes stroke survivors who are asked to move their fingers (or wrist or foot, etc.) deny that they have any movement. A concerned doctor might say, "Humor me, and give it a try," and sure enough, there is movement. Not much movement, but enough to apply **repetitive practice**, rewire the brain, and begin an upward spiral of recovery. Challenge feeds recovery. Recovery feeds on challenge.

- *Safe*: There are two reasons to stress safety:
  — Injuries are bad; everyone knows this, and everyone knows why. A simple slip and fall can lead to a broken bone, a hospital stay, a pressure sore, and even death.

— Injuries stop recovery. The threshold for an injury that stops recovery is much lower than anything that involves a hospital stay. A torn muscle, a sore back, or a bruise can slow or stop recovery efforts.

What Precautions Should Be Taken?

Inherent in designing an effective rehabilitation program is a commitment to new and challenging areas of physical experience. This is as true with stroke survivors as it is with athletes, musicians, dancers, and other individuals who use their bodies to express themselves, pursue their passions, and make their living. The trick for survivors is to make the rehabilitation efforts both challenging and effective while remaining safe. Consulting your doctor and involving physical, occupational, and other healthcare providers will go a long way in maintaining the safety/challenge dynamic.

EAT TO RECOVER

Diet has huge implications on so many levels for everyone. Diets impacts . . .

- The development and recovery from diseases like diabetes, heart disease, and diseases of the blood vessels
- The immune system
- Mental acuity
- Quality of life

The impact of diet on survivors is even larger than on the general population, because diet affects so many aspects of recovery. For instance, diet affects energy levels, physical performance, mood, cardiovascular health (stroke is a cardiovascular disease), and muscle strength. And, of course, diet affects weight. The less you weigh, the easier it is to move. The opposite is true, as well; the heavier you are, the harder it is to move. Weight gained is weight that has to be lifted during movement. The heavier a stroke survivor is over optimum weight, the more difficult the path to recovery. Stroke survivors tend to cascade toward weight gain. In some folks, stroke initiates a downward spiral that might look like this:

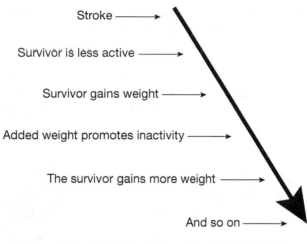

Stroke ⟶

Survivor is less active ⟶

Survivor gains weight ⟶

Added weight promotes inactivity ⟶

The survivor gains more weight ⟶

And so on ⟶

Downward pattern of weight gain in stroke survivors.

How Is It Done?

So what exactly is the correct diet for someone rehabbing from stroke? Lots of useful information in libraries, on the web, and from health professionals will provide all the specific diet suggestions you'll ever need. Here are a few basic dietary guidelines for anyone trying to improve physical performance:

- *Try to remain within your optimum weight.* It's a lot easier to lift your arm if it weighs 20 pounds than if it weighs 30 pounds. Your doctor can tell you your optimum weight. Weight beyond your optimum makes training after stroke difficult because extra weight is weight that has to be lifted, shifted, and held whenever you move. Also, unnecessary fat needs to be vascularized (blood vessels need to be manufactured by your body to feed the extra cells). This extra vascularization makes the heart have to work that much harder to pump that much more blood to these new vessels.

- *Choose quality carbohydrates.* Carbohydrates can be bad (processed) or good (unprocessed).

  — Processed (also known as refined or simple) carbohydrates like white rice, potato chips, pretzels, white bread, white sugar, candy, sodas, and so on, are digested and absorbed into the blood rapidly, which causes a rapid spike in blood sugar. The quick release of sugars puts stress on the system to quickly reduce blood sugar. The organ responsible for controlling blood sugar is the pancreas. The chemical it uses to decrease blood sugar levels is insulin. The pancreas and insulin do their job well. They do it so well that high blood sugar becomes low blood sugar after eating simple carbs. Folks eat again, often craving simple carbs, in an attempt to offset the loss of energy (caused by low blood sugar). Enough of these roller coaster rides of sugar levels and the pancreas becomes overwhelmed and cannot produce enough insulin. If that happens, diabetes can develop.

— Unprocessed (also known as unrefined or complex) carbohydrates like whole grain bread, brown rice, and whole fruits (apples, oranges, etc.) provide a much more gradual digestion of the carbohydrate, resulting in a much more gradual release of sugar. The slower the release of sugar, the better, because a gradual release can be better absorbed, stored, and used by the body.

- *Stay away from bad fats.* Bad fats include hydrogenated and partially hydrogenated fats. Hydrogenated fats are oils that are heated, and once they cool, stay solid at room temperature. Partially hydrogenated fats are oils that are heated, and are somewhere between solid and liquid at room temperature. Hydrogenated and partially hydrogenated oils are found in fried foods and are ingredients in pastries, chips, cookies, crackers, muffins, donuts, candy, and much of fast food. These bad fats are written in the ingredients list on a food package as hydrogenated vegetable oil, partially hydrogenated vegetable oil, or shortening.

- *Use good fats.* The flipside to the oil equation is increasing good fats in your diet. Good fats include extra virgin olive oil, cod liver oil, nut oil, flaxseed oil, and canola oil. Another important fat is fish oil. Fish oil has a near perfect ratio of the three important fatty acids: eicosapentaenoic acid (EPA), docosahexaenoic acid (DHA), and alpha-linolenic acid (ALA). Fish oil may help stroke survivors in two ways:

1. DHA and EPA may help to reduce swelling in the brain after stroke.

2. Fish oil helps overall function of the nervous system and is considered "neuroprotective" (a substance that protects the nervous system).

- *Good fats will actually lower the level of bad fats.* These good fats can have health-boosting qualities. High levels of good fats before a stroke decrease memory loss and disability after a stroke.

- *Eat a lot of fresh fruits and vegetables.* Fruits and vegetables have important vitamins, minerals, and amino acids (the building blocks of proteins).

Fruits and veggies should be eaten in a state that is as unprocessed as possible. Processed means cooked and/or combined with other ingredients. For instance, simply slicing a fruit or vegetable will reduce the amount of vitamins and minerals it has because some of the nutrient-rich juice is lost. Fruits and vegetables that are unprocessed and fresh will provide the greatest nutritional value. Fruits and vegetables help satiate your hunger, which keeps you from eating less healthy foods.

One habit that is essential to a healthy diet is simply reading the ingredients of what it is you eat. Reading the ingredients will lead to simple but profound questions like:

- "What is that ingredient?"
- "Why is that chemical in this food?"
- "How does this food compare to its whole (unprocessed) version?"

These questions inevitably lead to better dietary choices because they provide information about what you are eating, and help you to question why you eat what you do.

Buildup in the walls of arteries, the blood vessels that carry blood from the heart to all the cells in the body, is the cause of many strokes. This buildup is called plaque. High levels of a chemical called homocysteine can cause plaque buildup. People who have had a stroke have a tendency toward high blood levels of homocysteine. This may be a problem that is easily solved. Ask your doctor about the use of vitamin B12 to reduce levels of homocysteine. It is worth noting that high levels of homocysteine also increase your chance of disability after stroke.

Stroke can affect your ability to taste. Stroke can make foods taste weird, bad, or it can reduce your ability to taste at all. There is even a word for this change in the ability to taste after brain injury: *dysgeusia*. There may be a tendency to overcome the lack of taste by adding taste enhancers like salt, extra sauces and spices, or by frying foods. Be prudent and healthy with your choices as you attempt to make food palatable.

What Precautions Should Be Taken?

Inform your doctor about any major changes in your diet, even if they are considered healthy. For instance, switching to a vegetarian diet may be considered healthy but may not be appropriate for you at this time.

MAKE HOME MOVIES

Videotaping your recovery efforts can provide all sorts of information about your recovery. Researchers use all sorts of sophisticated and expensive tests to determine if a therapy is working. From brain imaging to computers that measure joint angles, researchers attempt to get the most accurate data possible. But at the end of the day, some of the most convincing information comes from simple videotape. Why is video so important? Because we humans are visual beings, and we believe what we see.

You can use the information that video provides to evaluate many different aspects of your recovery. Some of the questions to think about when reviewing your videotapes include:

- Is movement quality improving?
- Are movements performed faster but with the same or better coordination?
- Is walking more fluid and coordinated?
- Is there a reduction of tremor (shaking)?
- Is targeting (ability to move a body part into a space at which you are aiming) better?
- Are movements more symmetrical?
- Is a given task completed with more coordination and finesse?
- Are tasks performed better than before?
- Do any movements look incorrect?
- Do you seem to be in any danger when you move? Do you see that you are at risk for falling?

In the short term, video can provide valuable feedback about body position, timing, duration, and quality of movement, among many other aspects of recovery. First, you take a video of yourself performing a task, and then immediately watch the tape. As you view the tape, make a mental note on how you can improve in the future. Athletes use videotaping in this way all the time. A golfer will take a video of a swing and then watch the video and critique small components of the swing. This feedback allows you to view the task almost immediately, but, unlike viewing the task in a mirror, you can fully and objectively concentrate on the quality of movement. In this way, videotaping can provide short-term feedback.

Video can provide long-term feedback as well. Recovery tends to be very gradual. It is difficult for you to objectively view progress unless there is a way to review where you started. Once you see that you've improved, you'll be motivated to improve even more. Video delivers "Ah-ha!" moments as you realize that movements or tasks can now be accomplished that, just a few days (or weeks or months) ago, were impossible.

Audio recordings can be made to evaluate speech. Audio recordings may have advantages over video recordings of speech because the wide range of oral maneuvers that stroke survivors use to formulate words often look unco-ordinated but produce the best and most understandable speech. Audiotape will help you focus on the quality of your speech, rather than what it looks like. On the other hand, there may be times when you want to see the way your mouth is moving. There are two kinds of problems with speech that may result after stroke: aphasia and dysarthria. **Aphasia** is damage to the word-processing part of the brain. **Dysarthria** is a problem with the part of the brain that controls movement at the mouth. Someone with dysarthria may benefit from seeing how his or her mouth, lips, and tongue are moving on a video.

How Is It Done?

All you need is a video camera. A cell phone cam will do. Inexpensive and pocket-sized digital cameras can go wherever you go. Most computers can be rigged with an inexpensive video camera, which puts the video right on your computer. Digital video from your portable camera can be uploaded and organized onto your home computer, as well.

It may be helpful to take video from several different angles (front, side, back, etc.). Once a video is made, note where and when it was made. Use the same or similar environments, footwear, objects, and so forth, to make future comparisons more accurate. Keep the movements or tasks consistent through all your videos. This will help you compare "apples to apples." Focus on quality of movement more than speed, unless speed is essential to the task. Researchers will often test at two speeds: fast and self-selected (the speed at which you are most comfortable for that movement). When researchers and therapists test the movement of stroke survivors, they try to capture the best movement possible. They want the stroke survivor to try to perform the task as if he or she never had a stroke. When you are videotaping, it may help to first take a video of someone who has not had a stroke. Have them perform the same movement in an "ideal" way. Their movement can be analyzed with respect to your movement, and revealing comparisons can be made.

What Precautions Should Be Taken?

Do not compromise safety when videotaping. Because you may have to be the subject as well as the photographer, there may be wires, stands, or other equipment that can interfere with safe walking.

DON'T NEGLECT THE "GOOD" SIDE

"The squeaky wheel gets the grease." This is true with stroke survivors who often put much of their effort into training the "squeaky" limbs on the "bad" side. There are a lot of scientifically valid reasons to work on the "bad" side, but there are also good reasons to work with the "good" side of the body.

How Is It Done?

Here is an outline of reasons to work the "good" side:

- *Research has shown that stroke affects both sides of the brain and body.* Researchers really don't use the term "unaffected side." They use the term "less affected side." The fact is that both sides are affected by the stroke and can benefit from exercise and coordination training.

- *During parts of the recovery process, the "good" side is going to accept more of the responsibility of everyday life.* From dressing to driving, more is going to be asked of the "good" side. Since this side has a greater role, it needs more strength, flexibility, and coordination. For folks whose stroke affects their dominant side (e.g., the right side is affected for someone who is right-handed), new responsibilities are accepted by the nondominant (left) extremity. Some of the new skills will involve fine-dexterity activities like writing and grooming. For this reason, just to continue the activities of daily life, the stroke survivor needs to work on coordination of the less affected side.

- *The "good" side can be used to exercise in ways that the affected side cannot (in the short term).* For example, at some points in recovery, a cardiovascular workout may only be able to be accomplished by the less affected side because the "bad" side has a limited ability to move, but there is still cardiovascular benefit from letting the "good" side do all the work. This is not an invitation to concentrate recovery efforts only on the less affected side. Rather, "working with what you've got" provides a short-term strategy for doing all sorts of strengthening and cardiovascular training at any point during recovery.

- *When both sides are worked together, the affected side is going to fatigue much faster.* Once the "bad" side is too fatigued to work and needs time to rest, recovery efforts can continue by working with the less affected side.

Recovery from stroke often sets survivors on a course to a healthier overall lifestyle. For some people, it fosters an increased attention to health issues. For others, it provides a renewed focus on how their bodies move. This renewed focus on health will lead to working with your body—your whole body—which provides benefits to your health and recovery. Overall health and stroke recovery are intertwined and cannot be separated. Each depends on the other. Using the "good" side to promote overall health will also help recovery.

What Precautions Should Be Taken?

Remember: During the first ten days after stroke, using the affected side may decrease recovery of the affected side overall. Working the "good" side may be helpful for the reasons outlined earlier, but it is not recommended to use this strategy during the first ten days after stroke.

Working hard with the "good" side will challenge the heart and lungs in a way that would otherwise be limited. Because working the "good" side will encourage an increased intensity of exercises, you should inform your doctor of the intensity increase.

Lower-extremity exercises done by the unaffected side may place extra strain on the affected leg and foot, leading to falls and resultant injury. Keep this in mind when performing any exercises that challenge balance while standing.

GUIDE YOUR DOCTOR

While reading this book you may have found one recurring theme: "Push the issue." In all areas of stroke recovery, you should work to achieve, and expect, the most recovery possible. Recovery is best served when you and your caretakers always "push the issue."

Doctors, nurses, and therapists are used to the lowered expectations of the typical stroke survivor. They may assume that you have similar expectations. Stroke survivors can sometimes influence clinicians toward lowered expectations. Clinicians then use what they've learned to influence other stroke survivors. Each influences the other. (Note: For the rest of this section, doctor will mean whatever health-care provider you're talking to.) The bottom line is: Your doctor may not realize that you need to get better. Many doctors still believe that little or no recovery occurs after the subacute period. If your plan is to achieve as much recovery as possible, it is going to be unusual and unexpected. It is up to you to let your doctors know that you want to take your recovery as far as it will go, and that you want them on your recovery team. Doctors will be motivated to push the issue if you are motivated; both of your ambitions will feed off each other. Consider your relationship with your doctor a partnership dedicated to your recovery.

How Is It Done?

When you talk to your doctor about your recovery from stroke, keep it simple. Talk to your doctor about specific problems, issues, and thoughts. For instance, don't say something general like, "I want to move better." Instead, focus on more specific problems relating to movement deficits. For example, spasticity will often cause the hand to be postured in a tight fist. This will make the hand difficult to open and difficult to clean. Also, the nails become difficult to trim. Because of the strength of the fist, the nails begin to cut into the hand. This specific problem requires specific attention. In this case, you would tell your doctor that your nails are cutting into your hand, and that you want to be able to open the hand. The doctor then can provide a specific treatment that will target that specific problem.

As you discuss your recovery with your doctor, keep the following two goals in mind:

- *Convince your doctor that you are going to "push the issue."* You have made the decision to go forward, no matter what the naysayers claim and despite what your body is (sometimes) telling you. Let your doctor know that you need them to help you in this vision quest.

- *Talk to your doctor about the effectiveness and safety of the next series of treatment options in your plan.* That is, you have to let your doctor know what the short-term plan is. Focusing on the short-term portion of your plan will help retain your doctor's focus and enthusiasm.

Here are suggestions when visiting with your doctor:

- Bring a written list of questions.

- Bring a written list of goals.

- Bring an advocate (friend, family member, or caregiver) with you. Discuss with your advocate what you want to know and why you want to know it before the appointment, so if you forget a question, they can chime in.

- Bring a list of prescription and over-the-counter medications and supplements you are taking. Discuss how your medications might be affecting your recovery.

- Be prepared to take notes. Bring a pencil and paper or a tape recorder.

- Suggest that your doctor write a script (prescription) for occupational, physical, and speech therapy, if therapy is needed to achieve the next step in your recovery.

- Get feedback from the doctor on treatment options that you've researched and are thinking of implementing.

Keep two things in mind when choosing doctors:

- *Your primary doctor may not be knowledgeable about the cutting-edge recovery options* that you will need, from time to time, to continue progressing toward recovery. A physiatrist (see the section A Doctor Made for Stroke Survivors in Chapter 1) is a doctor who specializes in rehabilitation. Consider having your primary doctor refer you to a physiatrist. Physiatrists will be knowledgeable about the use of cutting-edge recovery options. He or she will also have specialized tools that will help you during your recovery quest.

- *Some doctors are not aggressive.* If the doctor you choose does not understand your ambitious plan, get another doctor. This is especially true for the specialists (neurologists and physiatrists) who will need to be on-board for your recovery plan to be successful.

What Precautions Should Be Taken?

Push the issue!

7 Spasticity Control and Elimination

SPASTICITY—THE BEAST UNMASKED

What Is It?

Spasticity is a disorder that is rarely fully explained to stroke survivors. Clinicians tend to describe spasticity in terms of its effect on muscles or body parts. For instance, they may say, "The stroke causes your hand to be tight," or they may say, "Your muscles are tightening because of the damage caused to your brain by the stroke." These explanations of spasticity are incomplete. You need the whole story. Without an understanding of the cause of spasticity, there is little chance of reducing spasticity. Spasticity reduction, like most of stroke recovery, comes from the inside out. Only stroke survivors can reduce their spasticity. Like so many other aspects of stroke recovery, stroke survivors "drive their own nervous system" toward recovery. Spasticity is a nervous system issue. Spasticity is caused by the brain's lack of control over muscles. Muscles are affected, but are not the cause.

How Is It Done?

How can spasticity be reduced or eliminated in a way that does not involve drugs or surgery? The only way to silence spasticity is to restore control of the spastic muscles to the brain. Using the **neuroplastic** process is the only way to restore control of the muscles. An understanding of spasticity will help you use the neuroplastic process to reduce spasticity.

Here is an explanation of spasticity that is scientifically correct and, hopefully, easy to understand:

How the brain controls muscles before stroke:

- Your brain tells your muscles when to contract (tighten, to help you move) and when to relax.

How the brain works after stroke:

- Stroke kills part of the brain responsible for control of affected muscles.
- The damaged part of the brain no longer "hears" those muscles.
- The brain no longer tells affected muscles when to contract or when to relax.

If your brain is not fully able to control your muscles, what makes them tight? Are the muscles acting alone? Or is something telling them to tighten?

How the spinal cord causes spasticity:

- Muscles constantly send signals to the spinal cord. Normally, the spinal cord sends those signals up to the brain.
- Because of the stroke, the brain no longer gets the messages sent from the muscles, so the brain no longer "hears" the muscles. Because of this lack of communication, muscles are under no brain control. Muscles hate being out of control because it means they may overstretch and tear (muscles tear easily).
- Since the brain cannot keep muscles from tearing, the spinal cord takes over the job.
- The spinal cord can only send out one message to muscles: "Muscles, contract!" The spinal cord is a poor brain, but it was not designed to be a brain. It was designed to be a "messenger boy" from brain to muscles and from muscles to brain. Spasticity is a bad thing, but without the spinal cord giving the "Muscles, contract!" command, those muscles would be flaccid (completely and utterly relaxed). Flaccid muscles can lead to tearing of the muscles, **subluxation of the shoulder, shoulder-hand syndrome**, and so on.

- Impulses from the spinal cord protect muscles by keeping them immobile.

  — *Good news:* The spinal cord protects that would otherwise be flaccid and at risk.

  — *Bad news:* The protection provided by the spinal cord leads to spasticity.

  — *More good news:* Spasticity can help you move, help keep muscles and bones strong. And, at least some messages are getting through to "bad side" muscles.

  — *More bad news:* Too much spasticity can cause a complete lack of movement. Very spastic muscles can turn into something other than muscle (connective tissue) and cause **contracture**.

The impulse that the spinal cord sends out to protect muscles is similar to a stretch reflex. An example of this is when a doctor tests reflexes with a reflex hammer. When the doctor hits you right below the kneecap, your knee extends. The knee extends whether you want it to or not. The movement of the leg kicking forward is called a *stretch reflex*. Stretch reflexes stop muscle tearing by instantly shortening muscles. Imagine if the doctor hit the knee over and over and never stopped. Spasticity can be viewed in a similar way. That is, spasticity is a repetition of reflexes.

What spasticity does:

- The spinal cord tells the muscles to contract (shorten).
- This command *is* spasticity.
- In a matter of a few days, spasticity permanently shortens some muscles.
- Shortened muscles perceive any lengthening as a threat of tearing.
- The muscle sends out an increased amount of "Help! I'm tearing!" messages to the brain and spinal cord. But the brain never "hears" the message because the brain was injured by the stroke.
- The spinal cord continues to send signals to the muscle to tighten.

Here is a representation of the process of spasticity in the stroke survivor:

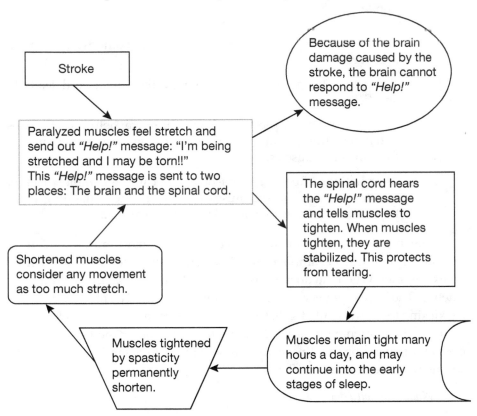

And around and around it goes: The muscle keeps saying "Help!" and the spinal cord says "Contract!" This process makes the muscle tighten even more, causing more "Help!" signals from the muscle. In some survivors, spasticity can continue during everything but the deepest stages of sleep. In most survivors, however, spasticity wanes before the survivor falls asleep.

What Precautions Should Be Taken?

None.

NEUROPLASTIC BEATS SPASTIC

The brain uses muscles to control movement. Muscles will contract and relax in a precise way to allow you to move fluidly. After stroke, the connection between brain and muscles on the "bad" side is broken. The "bad" side muscles may be under little (if any) control, and muscles hate being out of control. Since the muscles are no longer under control, they turn to the spinal cord for control. It is this relationship between muscles and spinal cord that is the core of spasticity. After a stroke, the brain can no longer protect the muscle from being overstretched and torn, so the spinal cord takes over and tells the muscles to stay tight, which protects them from being torn. Spasticity is a protection mechanism. The problem, of course, is that tight muscles make it difficult to move. No drugs, therapies, or modalities will permanently eliminate spasticity. They are all temporary; once they are withdrawn, spasticity returned. There is hope, however. Hiding in plain sight, the answer to the riddle of spasticity may be simple: Repetitively move the spastic muscles.

The Neuroplastic Model of Spasticity Reduction

Purging muscles of spasticity involves our old friend, **neuroplasticity**. The stroke kills the part of the brain that controls spastic muscles. But what if that was reversed? What if you could dedicate more brain to spastic muscles? That is the neuroplastic model of spasticity reduction. The idea is to use techniques that will give spastic muscles a larger part of the brain. When control of muscles is retaken by the brain, spasticity wanes. Muscle tightness will become less intense, which will, in turn, provide more control of movement. More control of movement will allow for a wider range of movement. A wider range of movement will allow the body to drive more changes in the brain. The more control the brain has over muscles, the more movement is available. The more movement available, the more brain changes can be driven, and so on.

The primary tool used to re-establish brain control over spastic muscles is repetitive practice. For instance, **constraint-induced therapy**, which uses a lot of repetitive practice, will often decrease spasticity. But your efforts to regain brain control over spastic muscles are not required to follow any standardized "treatment" or "protocol." Getting the brain to take responsibility for muscles requires using those muscles over and over (repetitively). These repetitive efforts should also be challenging—"nipping at the edges" of your current ability.

Put simply:

- Repetitive and challenging practice of spastic muscles reduces spasticity because . . .
  - Repetitive practice restores brain control over muscles
  - Restoring brain control over spastic muscles reduces spasticity

How Is It Done?

The downward spiral after stroke:

> Stroke → The part of the brain that controls muscles is damaged → The brain cannot control, or protect, muscles → The spinal cord protects muscles by making them tight → Muscles permanently shorten → Tight, shortened muscles make movement difficult.

The upward spiral after stroke:

> Repetitive practice rewires the brain → The brain regains responsibility for muscle control → The spinal cord gives control of muscles to the brain → Spasticity declines or is eliminated → Movement is made more normal.

The only way to permanently reduce or eliminate spasticity is by rewiring the brain to regain control over muscles. The same recovery options that promote brain rewiring will reduce spasticity as well. Increased movement and reduced spasticity are two sides of the same coin.

- As spasticity decreases, the ability to move improves.
- Improved movement chips away at spasticity.

Let's be clear about this: The neuroplastic model of spasticity reduction involves activating spastic muscle repeatedly. This is controversial among some healthcare workers. Many in healthcare were taught to not use spastic muscles. The reasoning was this: If you use spastic muscles you'll increase the strength of those muscles. If you strengthen spastic muscles, spasticity gets worse by strengthening the spastic pull. There are two problems with this thinking:

- Spastic muscles are weak. So even if you strengthened them, it would not necessarily be a bad thing.
- The brain will regain control over spastic muscle, thereby decreasing spasticity, but only if those muscles voluntarily move. Spastic muscles, when used in a repetitive way, increase their brain representation. That's the neuroplastic model of spasticity reduction.

Spasticity is not just bad because it affects muscles—spasticity also affects the brain. Animal research studies have shown that if a limb is immobilized (usually by strapping the limb to the body), the number of brain cells dedicated to that limb shrinks. This is exactly what happens to stroke survivors with spasticity. Their muscles are immobilized by spasticity. If the spastic muscles resume movement, the portion of the brain representing those muscles will get larger. As more brain power goes into those muscles, spasticity will subside.

Treatments that **physiatrists** and neurologists use can help you to rewire your brain to regain control over spastic muscles. These doctors have specialized training in treatments that reduce spasticity. Some drugs and other treatments provide temporary relief from spasticity. The temporary relief can allow for easier movement. The temporary relief may also help create an opportunity for the hard work of rewiring your brain.

Drugs used to reduce spasticity fall into two groups:

- Those given locally (injected directly into the spastic muscles) or administered into the fluid surrounding the spinal cord. These drugs affect only specific muscles.

- Those taken orally. These drugs will affect all the muscles in your body.

These drugs can reduce spasticity, which can:

- Improve movement
- Increase the potential of recovery
- Curb potential bone and joint problems
- Reduce pain
- Increase strength
- Reduce the risk of **contracture**
- Set the stage for neuroplastic change

Ask your doctor about these options. Remember, though, these medications will not address the underlying cause of spasticity (lack of control by the brain over muscles). No drug will replace the hard work needed to rewire your brain. The drugs and other treatments that temporarily reduce spasticity provide a window of opportunity for you to do the hard work of rewiring the brain.

The hard work comes in the form of:

- **Constraint-induced therapy**
- The use of **repetitive, task-specific massed practice**

- Some electrical stimulation (e-stim) treatments
- Some forms of **bilateral training**
- **Mental practice**

This list will grow with emerging research, so continue to explore the research and ask lots of questions.

What Precautions Should Be Taken?

Consultation with your doctors, therapists, and other health professionals will help direct your therapy so that spasticity reduction is achieved with a minimum of waste and a maximum of treatment effect.

You and your doctor may decide to use spasticity medications for reasons other than offering a window of opportunity for neuroplastic change. There may be other very good reasons for oral and other forms of spasticity medications. Reasons for continued use of systemic spasticity medications may include better mobility, less pain, better movement, and so on.

SPASTICITY, TONE, AND CONTRACTURE: EVEN CLINICIANS GET IT WRONG

Spasticity after stroke is often confused with tone and contracture, but they are different.

Confusion About the Terms Spasticity and Tone

Spasticity, and all the other muscles issues mentioned earlier, are often confused and conflated—even by clinicians. It is important to know the difference because they are

- Caused by different things
- Diagnosed differently
- Treated differently

How Is It Done?

If the muscle has

Tone: The muscle is normal. Muscle is easily moved. Evident, and measurable with electromyography (EMG), tone exists even in relaxed, "normal" muscle. The brain is doing its job controlling muscles well.

Spasticity: Muscles are stiff but moveable. The stiffness increases when the muscle is moved fast. Spasticity is said to be "velocity dependent"; the faster you extend (lengthen) the muscle, the more resistance you get. The part of the brain responsible for the spasticity is not doing its job.

Contracture: Muscles are not moveable. The muscle has become shortened. Although it is often confused for spasticity, it is not spasticity. It may be caused by spasticity, but it is not spasticity. Spasticity is a brain problem. Contracture is a muscle shortening problem.

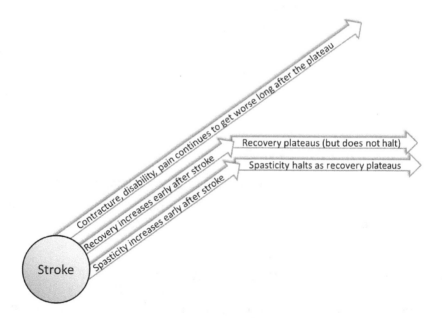

Although most clinicians think that spasticity after stroke is progressive (gets worse), this is only true in some survivors, and only before the plateau. Once the stroke has occurred, spasticity may (or may not) get worse. If it does get worse, the amount of spasticity will not get any worse once the survivor has plateaued. So, once the survivor plateaus, the spasticity plateaus. The reason clinicians think that spasticity gets worse over time is because they confuse spasticity with other problems brought on by the spasticity. Those things include pain, deformities, a loss of range of motion in the joint, and contracture. Spasticity does not get worse, but all those other things *do* get worse.

So, again, tone, spasticity, and contracture

- Are **caused** by different things.
  - — Tone: An intact brain
  - — Spasticity: The part of the brain that should be controlling the spastic muscles is not (because of the stroke)
  - — Contracture: Caused by spasticity, but now a muscle problem: The muscle is too short
- Are **diagnosed** differently
  - — Tone: feels normal when the muscle is extended
  - — Spasticity: The faster the muscle is moved, the more resistance there is to the movement
  - — Contracture: No matter the speed, there is the same amount of resistance
- Are **treated** differently
  - — Tone: No need to treat!
  - — Spasticity: See suggestions throughout this chapter
  - — Contracture: Serial casting and tendon lengthening (a surgery where the tendon is cut so the joint can be taken through its full range of motion)

What Precautions Should Be Taken?

A clinician well trained in diagnosing the difference between tone, spasticity, and contracture should be consulted to make this determination. In large rehabilitation hospitals there are often "spasticity clinics." These clinics are staffed with clinicians that know how to diagnose and treat spasticity and contracture.

SPASTICITY—JEKYLL AND HYDE?

What Is It?

In some ways, spasticity can be of temporary benefit as you move away from the "flaccid phase" of recovery.

Immediately after their stroke, some survivors are flaccid (limp) on the affected side. Nothing on the affected side can be moved under the survivor's own power. This is a scary time for survivors and their families. It is a cruel joke that stroke survivors are at their worst right after their stroke, when they are least able to understand and react to what has happened.

Research indicates that survivors who are flaccid for a year after their stroke can expect limited recovery. But some stroke survivors, who think they are flaccid, actually are not. Part of the problem is the words that are used to describe problems with movement. The word "paralyzed" is often used by folks who actually mean "hemiparetic." **Hemiparetic** means *weakness* on one side of the body, not paralysis. There are only two kinds of true paralysis after stroke:

- Flaccid paralysis (muscles do not contract—flex, fire, or move)
- Spastic paralysis (muscles are so tight with spasticity the survivor cannot move them)

These forms of paralysis are rare. Most stroke survivors fall into a broad category of "hemiparetic."

Some folks think this is a distinction without a difference, but they are wrong. Small amounts of movement can be used as a jumping-off point for much larger and more coordinated movement. So there is a huge difference between "no movement" and "small amounts of movement." Someone who is flaccid after a year has a poor prognosis for return of movement. Someone who has small amounts of movement has retained the brain-muscle connection, and growing that connection means there is potential for greater movement.

The *Brunnström* stages reveal that, as people recover from stroke, they go from a period of being flaccid and emerge into a period in which they are spastic. Having spasticity emerge is seen as a period of hope because muscles are finally able to contract. With the emergence of spasticity, often small amounts of **synergistic movement** occur.

Brunnström's stages state that after the flaccid period comes the emergence of spasticity. Can spasticity be viewed in some sort of positive light? The fact is that there are bad *and* good aspects to spasticity.

How Is It Done?

Spasticity is *bad* because it:

- Shortens muscles and other **soft tissue**, which can lead to permanent shortening (**contracture**)
- Positions joints abnormally, which makes limbs less functional
- Interferes with normal activities
- May cause pain
- May cause insomnia
- May cause deformities
- May cause poor weight gain (permanently contracted muscles burn a lot of calories)
- May cause pressure sores

Spasticity is *good* because:

- It is useful protection in cases of "**unilateral spatial neglect**" (when the stroke survivor is less aware or completely unaware of the affected side). For instance, in the arm and hand, spasticity will pull the limb across the body. This may be more desirable than the flaccid state, in which the limb is flopping around and fingers and arm are at risk for injury
- Is a step in the right direction from flaccid
- It may build bone strength (using **Wolf's law**), reducing the risk of osteoporosis
- It can be used to substitute for strength, allowing standing, walking, and gripping
- It sometimes makes transfers (e.g., going from sitting to standing) easier

- It may improve circulation, preventing blood clots and swelling
- It maintains muscle bulk

What Precautions Should Be Taken?

The emergence of spasticity can be seen as a positive sign in the overall arc of recovery. But once spasticity has been established, the next stage of recovery requires the reduction and eventual elimination of spasticity. As is true with much of stroke recovery: When one job is done, another begins.

GIVE SPASTICITY THE ONE–TWO PUNCH

Healthcare workers and stroke survivors sometimes make the mistake of thinking that spasticity in the arm is an arm problem or that spasticity in the leg is a leg problem. One thing is clear: Spasticity is a brain problem. Spasticity is a symptom of the brain damage caused by stroke. Spasticity is a protection mechanism that keeps muscles from being torn. The brain is no longer doing its job, so the spinal cord takes over the job of protecting muscles, joints, and other soft tissue (i.e., nerves, blood vessels, and the muscles themselves). The spinal cord sends out one message, over and over: "Muscles, protect yourself! *Tighten!*"

Many researchers believe that if enough of the right kind of **neuroplasticity** (brain rewiring) can occur, spasticity will be reduced; but there is a problem. For the neuroplastic process to start, you need the ability to initiate movements. If spasticity is too strong, movement becomes impossible. If neuroplasticity needs some movement, but the stroke survivor's limbs and fingers don't move because of spasticity, how do you jump start the process? For some stroke survivors, there may be a way.

There are three medications that can be used to target the specific muscles that are spastic: Botox, phenol, and alcohol. Together they are called "nerve blocks." Nerve blocks are usually administered by physiatrists or neurologists.

Botox

Botox has gotten most of its press because folks use it to get rid of wrinkles. The way it eliminates wrinkles is important in understanding how it works on spastic muscles. Lines in your face are created and accentuated by the

muscles that move your face around during frowning, squinting, and raising the forehead. A doctor can inject Botox, which temporarily paralyzes
these muscles and relaxes the muscle's pull on your face, allowing for fewer
wrinkles. Botox works on spastic muscles in the same way: It relaxes spastic
muscles.

If you hear the word "botulism" and immediately think of the food poi-
soning that makes people ill from eating food that has gone bad, you are right.
Botox is made from the same bacteria that causes botulism. That bacteria,
called *Clostridium botulinum*, gives off a substance that can paralyze muscles.
This substance is harvested from the bacteria to make Botox. Botox does not
contain the actual bacteria that causes botulism and does not give patients
botulism. Botox decreases the release of acetylcholine, which is a chemical
that allows a nerve signal to reach the muscles. In this way, it blocks nerve
impulses, like those that cause spasticity.

Phenol and Alcohol

These medications are injected directly into spastic muscles. Like Botox, they
temporarily weaken spastic muscles, thereby reducing spasticity. Prior to the
introduction of Botox these medications were used quite often. It should be
pointed out that both phenol and alcohol as spasticity-blocking agents are
significantly less expensive than Botox.

The combination of nerve blocks and exercise techniques used to initiate
movement can be effective in improving movement and permanently reducing spasticity. Botox is injected into tight muscles, and those muscles then
relax enough to unmask available movement. The idea is to allow for recovery
options that promote brain rewiring using movement that was impossible to
achieve prior to the administration of the nerve block. Each treatment with
nerve blocks usually relaxes the treated muscles for a few months. This treatment provides a window of opportunity to increase active (self-propelled)
movement. However, some nerve blocks can be administered more than once,
so multiple opportunities to increase movement exist.

There is a new treatment for spasticity reduction. It's called *hyaluronidase*
and, like Botox and both phenol and alcohol blocks, it is injected directly into
the spastic muscle. It shows promise, and has one unique advantage over other
nerve blocks: Hyaluronidase does not cause weakness in the injected muscles.
That's important because the other nerve blocks cause weakness. Normally a

survivor may be accustomed to having those muscles spastic and sometimes uses the spasticity to be more functional. For instance, a survivor may use muscles that are spastic around the knee to stabilize the knee during walking. When nerve blocks are injected, the survivor no longer has the spasticity to "lean on" and this can lead to less function and even falls. Hyaluronidase does not cause weakness and the muscle can be used. Here is a way to look at it: Nerve blocks make the spastic muscle weaker. Hyaluronidase "lubricates" the muscle so it is less stiff and more under the control of the survivor. This is an emerging therapy, and is not yet ready for widespread use.

How Is It Done?

There is a combination of treatments that, when used properly together, can jump start the process of spasticity reduction and encourage movement. This combination of treatments has three parts:

1. A nerve block is injected directly into spastic muscles.

2. (*This step may or may not be necessary.*) Electrical stimulation (e-stim) is used to help develop your ability to begin to move, even a little bit. The type of e-stim comes in one or more of three forms:

   • Cyclic e-stim

   • Electromyography (EMG)-based biofeedback e-stim

   • E-stim functional orthotics

3. Options that promote brain rewiring are used.

Example A: Robert cannot lift his affected foot because there is a lot of spasticity in the muscles that force the foot down (the calf muscles). He goes to his doctor. His doctor refers Robert to a physiatrist.

   • The physiatrist uses a nerve block to relax the calf muscles.

   • Once the spastic muscles are relaxed, Robert works hard to lift the foot. He also does a lot of stretching of the calf muscles. His relaxed muscles allow him to stretch more than he has been able to since his stroke, but Robert continues to have trouble lifting his foot, even a little, on his own.

   • Robert's physical therapist suggests cyclic (on, off, repeating) **electrical stimulation** on the muscles that lift the foot. Progress is slow, and since nerve blocks only last a few months, Robert suggests to his therapist that he try something he has read about: **electromyography (EMG)-based electrical stimulation.**

- The combination of the nerve block and the electrical stimulation works. Robert can lift his foot a little bit.

- Robert uses the newly gained bit of movement repetitively to build muscle and rewire his brain neuroplastically.

Example B: Kathy's hand is always flexed at the wrist and fingers. Spasticity is forcing her hand into a permanent fist, forcing the fingernails into the flesh of the palm. This causes cuts in Kathy's palm and makes her hand difficult to clean. Kathy goes to a neurologist.

- A nerve block is used to relax the muscles that are causing the wrist and fingers to bunch up. These muscles are located in the palm side of the forearm.

- Exercises are prescribed by an occupational therapist to stretch the muscles that were tight (the same muscles that got the nerve block) and strengthen the muscles that open the fingers and lift the wrist.

- Despite a lot of effort with the occupational therapist and at home, Kathy can only open her fingers a small amount.

- Kathy's therapist suggests she use an e-stim orthotic on her arm. The orthotic had been tried before with Kathy, but the e-stim was not strong enough to open her hand. But now the nerve block relaxed the hand enough for the e-stim orthotic to work.

- The combination of e-stim and practicing grasp and release allows Kathy to begin to open her hand on her own. Kathy notices that her "new" ability to pick up objects has helped not only her hand, but her elbow and shoulder as well.

Some doctors inject nerve blocks, but do not use any sort of intervention to build on the opportunity provided by the nerve block --- which is a mistake. Nerve blocks do not permanently eliminate spasticity. Instead, they create opportunities for spasticity to be permanently reduced. After treatment with a nerve block there should be some intervention to take advantage of the window of opportunity the drug presents.

A quick note about Botox. Some research has shown that electrical stimulation of the muscles that were injected with Botox can do two things . . .

1. Make the effect of Botox stronger, thereby requiring less medication. Botox is expensive. E-stim of muscles that are injected may require less Botox to be injected.

2. Lessen the time that injected Botox takes to "absorb" into the muscle. Without e-stim, Botox uptake is seven to ten days. With e-stim, Botox uptake is approximately two days.

So, direct e-stim to the target muscles will decrease the amount of Botox needed and increase the window of opportunity that the drug provides. *This is something that requires a medical doctor to approve.*

Here is a partial list of therapies that may be effective in conjunction with nerve blocks:

- Virtual reality

- **Repetitive practice**

- **Modified** and classic **constraint-induced therapy (mCIT, CIT)**

- Cyclic electrical stimulation

- Electromyography-based electrical stimulation with **biofeedback** (e.g., Mentamove, Neuromove™)

- Stretching programs aimed at the muscles treated

- Traditional occupational and physical therapy (which may include any or all of the therapies in this list)

There are two other treatment options for people with spasticity. One affects spasticity directly, and one affects the *symptoms* of spasticity:

- *Affecting spasticity directly:* Dorsal root rhizotomy (DR) or a selective dorsal rhizotomy is appropriate for people with profound spasticity. Spasticity can cause extreme pain, skin breakdown (bedsores), hygiene issues, contractures, and so on. A patient can experience all these, and have cognitive impairment. For this sort of patient, DR is a humane and reasonable option. DR involves the selective surgical severing of parts of the nerves that enter the spinal cord. These are the nerves that send messages from the muscle to the spinal cord. When these are cut spasticity is reduced or eliminated. DR has an upside and a downside. The upside is that it reduces or eliminates spasticity permanently. The downside is that it's not reversible, and it eliminates or reduces sensation from the corresponding nerves.

So if a DR is done to the nerves that represent the upper extremity, the patient would have diminished or absence of sensation from that extremity. This may be a reasonable trade-off for some patients with severe spasticity, especially those patients who are cognitively impaired.

• *Affecting the symptoms of spasticity:* Serial casting (SC) is a process where a cast is used to hold the joint in a particular position. The cast is applied, removed, and then reapplied (typically) every one or two weeks. Each cast more aggressively stretches the target muscles toward a more functional position. SC holds the muscle in a stretched position for long periods of time. SC is the only way that is clinically proven to increase the length of spastic muscles. SC is sometimes used together with nerve blocks.

What Precautions Should Be Taken?

Doctors, usually physiatrists or neurologists, will decide if you are an appropriate candidate for Botox treatment. After Botox is administered, adjunctive therapy can help foster the muscle relaxation that this treatment provides. Recovery options that involve electrical stimulation have contraindications and precautions. Discuss these with your medical doctor.

8 Motivation: Recovery Fuel

MEETING THE CHALLENGE OF RECOVERY

Here is an actual conversation I had with a stroke survivor:

> HER: Okay, Pete. You've been involved in stroke recovery research for a long time. What do you have that will help me recover use of my hand and help my walking?
>
> ME: I have good news and bad news. The good news is that I have a plan that will help you get the most recovery possible.
>
> HER: Great! I was hoping you'd say that!
>
> ME: The bad news is that you'll probably work harder than you've ever worked in your life.
>
> HER: Oh. I was hoping you could come up with something where I didn't have to work hard.

There the conversation died. She was unconvinced, and something I already knew was confirmed. The elephant in the room is that some stroke survivors don't want to work hard toward recovery. At least this survivor was honest.

Is it possible to maintain motivation when the going gets (*really*) tough? This is no idle question. Although many claim to be willing to change their lives in profound ways, if the stakes are high enough, more often than not, people choose not to change. Consider the stroke survivor who has never been in good physical shape, has never been an athlete, and

211

has never trained hard for physical gains. How is he going to magically transform into a "recovery machine?" How is he going to physically work harder than ever before?

Here are some thoughts about motivation:

- Maintaining motivation during the rigors of recovery is a discipline unto itself.
- It could not be simpler: People who stay motivated make progress.
- Motivation is essential to recovery, and if motivation is consistently maintained, it can drive recovery.
- Motivation is often the factor that has the most influence on recovery.
- Motivation is the core of recovery.
- Recovery from stroke is full of periods of incredible progress as well as disappointing lulls. Overcoming the slow periods and remaining focused is essential to the process of recovery.

People are motivated by a variety of different things. Here are a few quotes from stroke survivors regarding motivation:

- "I need to be independent. I don't want to rely on my family."
- "I have to get my hand and arm back. My weak arm has stopped me from things I love to do with my friends."
- "I want to be able to take care of my children (or grandchildren or great-grandchildren)."
- "I can't function with the constant fear of falling. I have to improve my balance and strengthen my legs."
- "I see my recovery as an adventure. I want to know how far I can go."
- "I don't want to walk funny. It's bad for business."

Here are some key words that may help you determine what motivates *you*:

Important

Essential

Embarrassing

Promotes independence

Sustains friendships

Allows childcare

Inspires fear

Saves (or helps you make) money

Makes you angry

A quick note about anger: In our society, anger is frowned upon, but anger is a powerful force that can be used to drive recovery. This is how Gandhi put it:

I have learned through bitter experience the one supreme lesson to conserve my anger, and as heat conserved is transmuted into energy, even so our anger controlled can be transmuted into a power which can move the world.

"Anger controlled" can be a powerful recovery tool.

Better Is Good

If you are willing to work hard, maybe harder than you've ever worked, you have the best chance of the highest possible level of recovery. Some survivors feel that the challenge of recovery is one of the defining moments in their lives. Accepting the challenges of recovery can make the difference between simply reclaiming something lost and embarking on a new adventure toward uncharted personal growth. Don't give up; don't give in. Recovery is full of ups and downs. Expect them to happen, and move on.

How Is It Done?

Motivation is tied to your personal aspirations, ambitions, and dreams. What motivates you toward recovery also depends on what you are unwilling to surrender. What you want to do and what you want back are powerful internal motivators. But if you do need inspiration from the outside, there are plenty of resources for that. Motivational stories can be found on the Internet, in books, movies, plays, and within one's faith. Books and movies can offer suggestions, and they can provide an opportunity to "experience" someone else making mistakes and finding solutions. In a word, these stories can *inspire*. The books and movies you choose do not have to be stroke specific. They can be stories about athletes, mountain climbers, war heroes, or anyone's story of survival and triumph.

Here are some other ideas for remaining motivated:

- *Recovery takes positive reinforcement.* Celebrate the small successes.
- *Turn recovery into a competition.* Successful athletes always compete against themselves.
- *Make recovery a social activity.* Your success can be fostered with the help of others, even if they are not stroke survivors.
- *Look for intensity of experience during recovery.* The intensity of the experience will help ingrain what is being learned.
- *Fall in love with the process of recovery.*
- *Have a recovery plan that includes measurable goals.* Success should be measured.
- *Make recovery efforts a part of your everyday schedule.*

The challenge of recovery is at once tenuous, difficult, fraught with frustration, and full of fits and starts. But like a four-wheel-drive vehicle plowing through banks of snow, hard work can compensate for much of the difficult terrain. Researchers are just beginning to unravel the riddle of recovery. The secret seems to be obvious: Recovery takes a tremendous amount of hard and sometimes frustrating work. Hard work drives cardiovascular and muscular strengthening. Hard work goes into planning and stroke recovery research. Hard work powers through plateaus and forges the neuroplastic process.

What Precautions Should Be Taken?

The often uncharted territory involved in hard work requires the aid of a doctor and other healthcare professionals to make the journey toward recovery a safe one.

BE A CAVEMAN

Nothing is forcing you to recover, and that just may be the problem. Archeologists make their living describing how our distant ancestors lived. They have found many skeletons of early humans with bone fractures, amputations, and skull trauma. Archeologists have also found evidence of arthritis, as well as an assortment of other injuries and illness. In many cases, these early humans survived their injuries. Human beings can have a stroke at any age. Many types of animals are known to have strokes. It can be assumed that these distant ancestors also had strokes. If a member of a tribal community had a stroke, his or her "therapy" would be ferocious. *Survival* of both the tribe and survivor would dictate their "caveman therapy." Efforts toward recovery would focus on walking because these early humans were hunter-gatherers and they needed to move quickly in search of food. Stroke survivors would have had to learn to feed themselves or go hungry, toilet or get bacterial infections, and walk or get left behind. Sheer survival dictated the tremendous amount of energy they put into their recovery efforts. Their rehabilitation would flow organically from what they knew they had to do.

No doubt, their recovery from stroke would be physically demanding, but they would have been used to huge amounts of hard physical work. Every day of their prestroke lives was a struggle for food and against the elements and beasts. Walking long distances, hunting, hut building, tool making, rudimentary sewing, foraging, and so forth, would have made these humans tough beyond modern understanding. In that sense, stroke survivors today are at a disadvantage. We've gone soft. Are we able to channel the toughness that hides deep in our shared DNA?

Along with a physical toughness, these ancestors would have had another advantage: They were forced to recover. No other member of the tribe would be able to speak as loudly as the survivor's own inner voice. "I want to *survive*." The end result of this raging for recovery would be more recovery than similar stroke survivors experience today. Much of this concept is covered in research under the term, **task-specific training**. Research has found that:

- If you practice a movement, you might get better at that movement.

- If you practice that same movement as part of a real-world task, you can expect more recovery.

- If you practice the movement within a real-world environment that is important to you, you can expect even more return of movement.

- If you practice a task that is vital to you, you will get the most return of movement.

The more vital the task is, the more you will be driven toward recovery. Early humans would have viewed almost everything they did, every day of their lives, as vital. Their tasks were more than just important: They were *essential* to survival. Their bones whisper the secret of recovery: *Work on recovery as if your life depends on it.*

How Is It Done?

Some stroke survivors use something close to this "caveman therapy." People who obtain the best recovery from stroke tend to be people who *have* to get better. Their life goals dictate that they must recover. They challenge themselves in ways that other stroke survivors don't. Driving their recovery are passions like independence, career, or essential hobbies like playing the piano, painting, or shooting pool. These modern-day "cavemen" and "cavewomen" are rare. They reclaim their passions because *their lives depend on it*.

The most effective clinical therapies mimic this recovery strategy. These therapies attempt to *force* recovery in one way or another. They are designed to cajole, prompt, and encourage, but they are, in the end, artificial. Researchers have been obsessed with designing artificial motivation. They try virtual reality, video gaming, and an assortment of other gizmos and tricks, but there is no substitute for that feeling from which recovery flows. What is it that you love? What in your life *must* you do? What do you have left to accomplish? Focus on these activities to unleash your inner caveman.

What Precautions Should Be Taken?

If skiing is your passion and you need to get back on your skis, don't just strap them on and head for the mountain. Include your doctor, therapists, family, and friends in your plans, and train safely as you move toward your goal. You are not a caveman. Your responsibility to your own recovery requires that you stay safe.

WHEN HELP HURTS

Life's day-to-day challenges present opportunities to work on recovery. Think about the devices you use to improve your life. Consider reducing any form of assistance that is not essential to safety and/or independence. Doing so will open up a world of productive struggle.

Assistive devices (ADs) and the broader term, **adaptive equipment**, are names for rehabilitation gear that:

- Makes your life easier
- Makes you safer
- Helps you be more independent in your daily life

Examples of these devices include:

- Specialized eating utensils
- Wheelchairs
- Reachers
- Leg lifters
- Zipper and button aids
- Writing aids
- Ambulatory aids (canes, walkers, etc.)
- Splints (ankle-foot orthoses, hand splints, etc.)

Assistive devices can promote independence, make your life easier, and make everyday living safer, but they may have a downside, too. These devices can make tasks that should be a challenge, easier. Doing without an AD can promote recovery. The challenge in everyday tasks is important to the process of recovery from stroke. It is worthwhile to weigh all the advantages of the AD, with special consideration regarding safety issues.

The typical medical model assumes that recovery from stroke is best served by making you safe, comfortable, and making life as easy as possible. *"Treat 'em and street 'em"* is often the mantra, and if "streeting 'em" requires a few helpful ADs, well then why not? There are actually good reasons for thinking this way. The stroke survivor, his or her family, and the insurance company decide the speed at which survivors are pushed through the system. Simply, the goal is to get you as independent as possible in the shortest amount of time. Part of this effort involves providing the necessary AD to speed up the process, but there are points in the arc of recovery where you should question the need for individual ADs. Keep in mind that an AD can mask the fact that you can do without the device. With every AD you use, you are asked to do less and are discouraged from doing more. Attempting less generally means less recovery. An ongoing and thoughtful evaluation of the necessity of all ADs is wise.

Consider pens with a built-up barrel. These "fat pens" have been used by stroke survivors for the same reason small children use oversized pencils: The fatter a writing utensil, the easier it is to control. When you use an oversized pen, you require less finger control. This continual lack of challenge reduces the chance of ever gripping regular pens and pencils. Coordination and dexterity are challenged less. The fine-motor aspect of gripping is not challenged, so all the tasks that require the same sort of grasp will suffer. Larger utensils should be used temporarily as you progress toward more challenging grasping tasks, but many survivors use these aids for the rest of their lives.

If the AD does not impact safety, then eliminating it becomes a decision based on its relative necessity versus the therapeutic value of not using it.

Here are two other ADs that should be reconsidered:

- Hand splints immobilize the joint of the forearm, wrist, hand, and fingers. There is no proof that splints improve movement or reduce **contracture**. Splinting eliminates the use of muscles that control the splinted joints. Immobilizing joints in this way may reduce the amount of brain dedicated to those joints. This causes a sort of "bad **neuroplasticity**." This reduces the amount of brainpower to those same joints, muscles, and movements that you're trying to recover. Some splints, especially off-the-shelf splints, can actually damage the joints in the hand by forcing the hand into unnatural positions. This can cause small tears in the joints of the hand and fingers.

- An **ankle-foot orthosis (AFO)** stabilizes the ankle and raises the foot during walking when the leg is swinging forward. The AFO makes walking easier, but less is being required of the foot and leg. The foot is no longer being asked to lift (dorsiflex) at the ankle. Also, less is required in terms of coordination of the entire "bad" leg and foot. There are good reasons for using AFOs, including important safety issues. However, if your doctor agrees and if walking can be done safely, the extra effort may pay off in:

  — Strengthening of the muscles that lift the foot

  — Increased coordination during lifting the foot

  — Strengthening of the muscles stabilizing the ankle

  — A larger area of brain cells dedicated to the ankle (**neuroplasticity**)

  — Increased ability to move the ankle

  — More challenge toward normal coordination of the entire "bad" leg and foot

Note: Do not end the use of splinting or an AFO without the consent and sanction of your doctor. Ending use of an AFO can lead to falls.

How Is It Done?

There are two broad ways to gradate the use of an assistive device (AD):

- Increasing or decreasing the *time* the device is used
- Increasing or decreasing the *type* of device, so there is more or less assistance

Some examples of gradation of dosage include:

- Choosing to begin to use the AD
- Increasing the amount of time that you use the AD
- Reducing the amount of time that you use the AD
- Ending the use of the AD

Some examples of gradation of type include:

- Examples of gradation of the amount of support used for walking
  — A walker (a lot of support)
  — Hemi-cane
  — Quad cane
  — Straight cane (a little support)
  — No walking aid (no support)
- Examples of gradation of aids used to lift the foot and stabilize the ankle
  — Ankle-foot orthosis
  — Ankle brace or ankle stabilizer (e.g., Aircast)
  — Flexible (e.g., Neoprene) ankle wrap
  — High-top athletic shoes
  — Shoes
  — Walking barefoot
- Decreasing the size of a "build-up" (widening the circumference) on a writing or eating utensil
- Reducing the use of or eliminating elastic shoelaces, buttoning, and zipping aids

This list represents just a few of a long and growing list of ADs used by stroke survivors. Occupational and physical therapists can provide a full list of available ADs.

What Precautions Should Be Taken?

The safety implications of ending your relationship with ADs can be enormous.

If the AD does impact safety, then a much more vigorous and thoughtful consideration must be taken. Ending usage of some ADs has the potential of putting the stroke survivor in danger. Consult with your doctor regarding ending use of any AD or splint. *Do not end the use of splinting or an AFO without the consent and sanction of your doctor.*

Also, it may be that you are not using an AD that you should be using. An AD can promote safety, independence, and/or promote recovery. New ADs are being developed and put on the market every day. ADs may provide efficiency and safety. They can also be an interim step on your road toward recovery. Some ADs have no downside and contain great benefits. For instance, grab-bars in the bathroom keep you safe in slippery areas, where challenging balance is dangerous.

RECONSIDER MEDICATIONS

Rule One: DON'T EVER STOP TAKING MEDICATIONS OR CHANGE DOSAGES WITHOUT DISCUSSING IT WITH YOUR DOCTOR!

Rule Two: DON'T EVER STOP TAKING MEDICATIONS OR CHANGE DOSAGES WITHOUT DISCUSSING IT WITH YOUR DOCTOR!

Rule Three: SEE RULES ONE AND TWO.

Drugs affect your recovery. Drugs include all medications that are prescribed, over-the-counter, or in foods (e.g., caffeine). Drugs affect everyone physically, emotionally, and/or mentally. Stroke survivors have the extra burden of trying to figure out how their medications affect their recovery efforts.

Therapists have always viewed their patients' medications as a mixed blessing. Consider antispasticity pills. They reduce spasticity, which helps make movement easier. Therapists like that movement is made easier, but these drugs are designed to relax *all* muscles. Because they affect all muscles, they tend to make patients tired. Tired patients cannot put their full mental and physical effort into their recovery. Pain pills, psychotropic medications (drugs that affect the mind), sleeping pills, and other drugs can have similar (tiring and/or unmotivating) results. Drugs can help or hurt your recovery. In fact, from one day to the next, the same medication may be a benefit and then a detriment. Consider narcotic pain medications. On Monday it may be too painful for you to move without the medication, so the drug is beneficial to recovery. On Tuesday you have little pain, but the medication has made you so tired that you can't focus on your therapy.

Sometimes adding a new medication clearly helps recovery. A stroke survivor, here called "Tim," has excruciating pain in his affected arm. Tim has what is called *shoulder-hand syndrome*. This is a form of **reflex sympathetic dystrophy (RSD)**, a problem in up to 25 percent of stroke survivors. The arm is so painful that Tim can't move it. Tim's primary doctor suggests Tim see a physiatrist. The physiatrist correctly diagnoses his pain and gives Tim a new medication that dramatically decreases the pain. This means Tim can finally move his arm in relative comfort. Efforts toward recovery can then begin.

The decision of which drugs should and should not be used is best left between you and your doctor.

How Is It Done?

So how do you go about reconsidering medications? The best way is called the "brown bag medication review." The idea is you throw all your medications in a brown paper bag.

In the bag should be . . .

- All prescription medicines (including pills and creams)
- All over-the-counter medicine taken regularly
- All vitamins and supplements
- All herbal medicines

All medications are placed on the counter in the exam room. The physician or pharmacist, with your help, decides which meds to keep, which to pitch, and which dosages to tweak. Some doctors estimate that if this review of meds is done, about 50 percent of the time the meds will, in some way, be wrong.

During the brown bag review, the following is also provided:

- Tips for safe and effective medication use
- Answers to your questions about medications

Once the whole thing is figured out, you are given a card that has all the medication information on it. This information would be available for you to review, and for you to hand to doctors, dentists, and others who may need to know your medications at a glance.

What Precautions Should Be Taken?

Again, *never* discontinue medications or change dosages without discussing it thoroughly with your doctor!

THIS JUST GOT *REAL*: PSYCHOLOGICAL ADJUSTMENT AFTER STROKE

What Is It?

Although not every survivor has psychological problems after stroke, many do. Sometimes those problems are

- Direct (because of the damage to the brain)
- Or indirect (because the stroke created such havoc in the survivor's life)
- Or, most likely, both direct and indirect

Direct damage cause by the stroke: Damage to the brain causes psychological and emotional changes. Although the mechanisms are not well understood, stroke in one area of the brain can cause disturbances in many other, distant parts of the brain. For instance, a survivor may have a stroke on the outside of the brain (closer to the skull). However, that injury often affects deeper structures in the brain that control anxiety, depression, emotional swings, anger issues, and fatigue.

Indirect damage to your life: Stroke is not just traumatic to the brain—it is traumatic to your life! So, while the actual brain damage may or may not have a psychological effect, the stroke inevitably creates problems that can challenge the survivor psychologically. These challenges can include changes in employment, relationships, independence (and on and on). They can create emotional and mental problems that can, at certain points in the arc of recovery, seem insurmountable.

Because of all these emotional stressors, all these normal psychological and social responses to stroke may slow physical recovery.

How Is It Done?

There is much less research on psychological adjustment than there is on physical treatment. The trick is to find the combination of your own efforts and supportive assistance that works for you. Each person will have their own strengths to draw upon. And each community will have its own set of resources available.

Some powerful self-care practices to boost your recovery efforts are:

- Spending time with friends
- Meditation
- Music and/or singing
- Spirituality
- Artwork or visiting museums
- Stroke support groups or discussions with other stroke survivors
- Home exercise centering time
- Guided imagery
- Yoga and/or breathing practices
- Time in nature
- Gardening
- Relaxed play time with children
- Relaxed play time with animals
- Nourishing meals
- Water therapy (classes or baths!)

Physiatrists (rehabilitation physicians) can support your efforts by referring you to:

- **Physical therapists and physical therapy assistants** can give you exercise routines that will be the most efficient use of your rehab energy and inspire you to keep exercising, which will improve your mood and *increase* your energy.

- **Speech therapists** can not only help you with improving your speech skills, but are also trained to assist cognitive rehabilitation, which can enhance your ability to plan and participate in your recovery program.

- **Psychologists** can help you form new patterns of thinking, and can educate you and your family about stroke issues and responses to life-changing events.

- **Occupational therapists and occupational therapy assistants** can help to improve quality of life by working with individual goals and skills for daily activities.

- **Social workers** help you to find the community resources that best suit your individual needs.

Precautions

Be sure to get enough rest. Make time to do what you love! Focused hard work is more satisfying and efficient if it is balanced by relaxation and fun. Be open with family and caregivers about any emotional issues that you're dealing with.

Be careful with expectations. Survivors sometimes confuse letting go of rigid expectations with giving up. Lack of expectation can lead to lack of effort, but too much expectation can lead to increased anxiety, frustration, and/or depression. Doing your best (including setting up social support) is the best way to increase recovery success and satisfaction.

FIGHT FATIGUE

Severe fatigue affects up to 70 percent of stroke survivors. Many survivors consider fatigue to be the worst symptom caused by the stroke. Post-stroke fatigue creates a downward spiral of disability. The more fatigue, the less effort is made toward cardiovascular and muscle strengthening. Decreased levels of exercise lead to weight gain, which leads to greater effort needed to move. This, in turn, leads to more fatigue, which leads to less exercise . . . and the spiral continues. Fatigue impacts many aspects of a stroke survivor's life, not the least of which is recovery. It goes without saying that, if you are too tired to fully engage in your recovery effort, less progress will be made.

There are many reasons for fatigue after stroke, including:

- Rehabbing in places that are typically noisy (primary hospitals, rehab hospitals, skilled nursing facilities, etc.). This allows for less quality sleep. Sleep is essential to recovery. See the section Horizontal Rehab: Good Sleep = Good Recovery in Chapter 5 for more information on the importance of sleep to recovery, as well as strategies to get adequate sleep

- A lot of tiring effort toward recovery

- Everyday activities use about twice the energy than they did prior to the stroke

- Survivors have about half the cardiovascular (heart and lung) strength compared to prior to the stroke

- Survivors have about half the muscle strength on the affected side compared to prior to the stroke

- Stress from life after stroke saps energy and makes sleeping more difficult

- Prescribed medications often add to fatigue

In some stroke survivors, the following may also cause, or add to, fatigue:

- Pain

- Depression

- Living alone

- Living in an institution

- Having trouble speaking or understanding

How Is It Done?

Here are some ideas and strategies to increase energy after stroke:

- *Get decent sleep.* Strategies to sleep better after stroke can be found in the section entitled Horizontal Rehab: Good Sleep = Good Recovery in Chapter 5.

- *As unbelievable as it may seem, exercise actually reduces fatigue*, even in the short term. Yes, exercise fights fatigue!
- *Increase your muscular strength.* The more stored strength your muscles have, the less fatigue you will experience.
- *Increase your cardiovascular strength.* The more stored energy your heart and lungs have, the less fatigue you will experience.
- *Meditate.* Stress saps needed energy. Meditation can reduce stress.
- *Reconsider your medications.* Some medications reduce energy. These medications can include psychotropic (drugs that affect the mind) and spasticity medications. On the other hand, other medications are stimulants. These drugs increase energy, at least in the short term. (Warning: Do not ever stop taking medications or change dosages without discussing it with your doctor!)
- *Proper nutrition can increase energy.* Eating refined carbohydrates (white breads, pastries, rice, pasta, donuts, bagels candy, soda, etc.) can reduce energy. Fresh fruits and vegetables and lean protein choices can increase energy.
- *Drink plenty of water.* Dehydration saps energy. As people age, their sense of thirst decreases, so drink water even when you aren't "dying of thirst."

What Precautions Should Be Taken?

All of the suggestions for fighting fatigue should be done under the supervision of your doctor. There are many medical reasons for fatigue, from dehydration to diabetes, and from pain to depression. It is essential that the underlying cause of fatigue be determined.

WALKING YOUR WAY TO BETTER WALKING

As obvious as it sounds, the best way of improving the quality of walking is to walk. The act of walking uses some of the most progressive concepts in recent rehabilitation research. For instance, one of the techniques researchers use to promote robust recovery is called **task-specific training**. This means training for recovery within the context of a valued task. There are few tasks more valued than walking. Walking also involves another buzz concept in rehab research: **repetitive practice** (the same movement is repeated). Researchers believe repetitive practice is essential to relearning a skill. Another cutting-edge concept in stroke rehabilitation is adding a **rhythmic** component. Walking is inherently rhythmic. Walking also involves another rehabilitation concept that researchers are keen on: **bilateral training**. Bilateral training involves having the two legs communicating with each other. Researchers believe that the two arms and two legs communicate with each other in two ways:

- The limbs communicate through the brain.
- The limbs communicate directly, right through the spinal cord, without the brain involved.

So walking brings together four advanced concepts:

- Task specificity: This involves practicing exactly what is to be learned.
- Repetitive: This involves doing the same movement over and over.
- **Rhythmicity**: This involves adding a beat. Walking itself supplies the beat.
- Bilateral training: This is where the two legs communicate directly. During bilateral training, the "good" limb can make the "bad" limb move better and faster.

Walking may just be the best exercise available. Walking:

- Is "low impact," so it puts little stress on the joints
- "Banks" energy for the heart and lungs
- Burns calories and controls weight
- Controls blood sugar
- Increases mental agility
- Decreases the chance of blood clots in the legs, which reduces the risk of another stroke
- Builds muscle
- Improves balance and may decrease falls
- Increases bone strength

. . . and much more.

How Is It Done?

There are a lot of ways to stay safe while pursuing an aggressive walking program. Proper orthotics, such as an **ankle-foot orthosis (AFO)**, and appropriate walking aids, such as canes and walkers, can be discussed with your doctor and physical therapist. If, however, you are not yet ready to walk without support, there are still options (beyond wearing a gait belt and having therapists help you). All of the following are done under the care of a physical therapist:

- *Treadmill training (TT)*: This can provide the safety and comfort of walking indoors with the added safety benefit of providing "endless parallel bars." Treadmill training has inherent risks that can lead to falling. See the section Train Well on a Treadmill in Chapter 2 for full details on treadmill training.

- *Partial weight-supported walking (PWSW)*

  — *PWSW on a treadmill*: You are partially supported by a harness. The harness can be raised to reduce the amount of weight you're carrying. The harness can also be lowered so that you are carrying your full weight, but the harness catches you if you fall. This allows you to challenge your balance without risk of falls. The product usually associated with this type of training is called the LiteGait®.

  — *PWSW over ground*: This system is the same as the treadmill version except you walk over flat ground. Products that fall into this category include the Biodex Unweighing System, the NeuroGym® Bungee Walker, and the LiteGait®. Contact a physical therapist or local rehabilitation hospital to find facilities in your area that provide PWSW.

- Researchers have found great results with a new kind of gait (walking) therapy. It is called **speed-dependent treadmill training**. It is a simple idea; your walking will get better and faster if you practice walking faster. When it comes to walking, speed is good. Research suggests that increased walking speed has a positive effect on attention, disability, mortality, future health status, confidence in balance, fear of falling, falls, where discharge will be, chance of hospitalization, and medical costs. Walking faster improves the quick movements needed to control balance, which translates into smoother and more efficient walking. Speed-dependent treadmill training has been used to double the walking speed of study participants.

What Precautions Should Be Taken?

Walking is one of the most natural movements humans perform, but a walking regimen designed to improve the quality of gait takes more physical and mental effort than leisure walking. Because this type of walking regime is more intense than leisure walking, make sure to talk to your doctor and therapist prior to incorporating therapeutic walking into a total rehabilitation plan. If you are able to walk without aid, do so with safety in mind. Your doctor and therapist will provide the medical and physical limits that should be observed.

THE YOUNG ADULT STROKE SURVIVOR (YASS): DRIVEN TO RECOVER

First, a question: What is a *"young"* adult stroke survivor (YASS)? Survivors can have their stroke at any time, even before birth (called an *in utero* stroke). A stroke early in life usually has a more profound imprint on the brain than a stroke later in life. The difference between an adult stroke and a stroke in children can be summed up in one word: *architecture.*

- *Stroke in adulthood: A normal architecture, altered.* Imagine building a new house. You build a good foundation, a solid frame, a strong roof, and so on. You put in the plumbing, electrical, and walls. Your new house is done. Then one day you have an accident! You back your car into the corner of the house. That part of the house needs to be fixed. The foundation is still there, the solid frame still exists in most of the house, the roof is still good; plumbing, wiring, everything is still good. You only need to fix that one room.

  — *A stroke in adulthood* affects a normally developed brain. The size and location of the stroke determines what skills are lost.

- *Stroke in childhood: An altered architecture.* Now imagine your neighbor builds a house, but he's not a very good builder. The foundation is uneven and the frame is crooked. Everything that is built around the foundation and frame is affected by the poor basic architecture of the building. To "fix" the house would require starting from scratch.

  — *A stroke in childhood* affects how the brain *develops*. The brain in childhood is a blank slate. Neurons (nerve cells in the brain) haven't "decided what they want to be when they grow up," and whatever is imprinted on that blank slate affects the way the brain develops. Children have an immense amount of brain plasticity available to them. After stroke, children often do amazing things, given the amount of brain injury they have. There are classic examples of children who have a complete hemisphere (half of their brain) destroyed by stroke. In an adult, such a stroke would institutionalize the person for the rest of his or her life, but some children survive and thrive with half a brain. They are able to learn to read, write, have a sense of humor, be productive, and enjoy life. So it is unfair to describe the brain after a childhood stroke as having "poor architecture." In fact, it could be considered "excellent architecture" given the amount of brain damage they have.

The impact of stroke before the brain is fully developed is much different than the impact of stroke after the brain is fully developed. The process of recovery in the two is very different as well. In fact, it is only in the adult brain that there is truly "recovery." In childhood stroke becomes a part of development.

The purpose of this section, and, in fact, this book, is to aid in *recovery*. Therefore, the "young" end of the spectrum will be defined as "after the brain is fully developed." But when is the brain fully developed? That is, when is someone biologically an adult? We know that the frontal lobes, responsible for impulse control, are not fully developed until around the 25th year. *Bottom line*: The young end of the spectrum is 25 years old.

The "old" end of the spectrum is also difficult to define. Somebody may be 50 years old, have had a stroke, and also have a number of other illnesses, as well. On the other hand, somebody may be 75 years old and have had no significant illnesses in their life except for the stroke. Typically, however, the upper age limit for a young adult stroke survivor (YASS) is 55 years old.

Definition of a YASS:

- A survivor of stroke between the ages of 25 and 55.

Some notable statistics about YASS:

- 15 percent to 20 percent of all strokes are in people under the age of 55.
- 30 percent of strokes are in people under the age of 65.
- The risk of stroke doubles for each decade after age 55, but the number of strokes is rapidly increasing in people between ages 15 and 34.

It is believed that the increase is due to a rise in obesity and associated problems like diabetes, high blood pressure, and lipid disorders.

• Stroke is actually decreasing among older adults, but it is increasing among younger people. This trend has held steady since the mid-1990s.

How Is It Done?

YASS have many advantages over older survivors in the quest for recovery. It may be more easily understood like this: YASS *don't* have many of the *disadvantages* that older survivors have.

YASS can work harder on recovery. They have the ability to put more effort into recovery, and effort is vitally important to recovery. Effort not only helps the heart, lungs, and muscles to get stronger, but effort drives changes in the brain.

There are other advantages young stroke survivors have. For instance, they . . .

• Have a better chance of surviving a stroke

• Are in better shape. Younger survivors naturally have stronger cardio-vascular (heart and lung) and muscle strength

• Usually have fewer other diseases (besides the stroke) than older survivors

• Have more physical resources to draw from. This means that a deficit in one area can be overcome more easily in a younger stroke survivor than an older survivor

  — Consider a vision problem sometimes seen after stroke: *hemianopsia*. Hemianopsia is a "visual field cut" where the stroke survivor can only see one side of his or her field of vision. The side the survivor can see is the same as the unaffected (good) side of the stroke. The side he or she *can't* see is the *"bad"* side. In an older stroke survivor, it would be more difficult to compensate for this visual field cut. The younger survivor typically has better neck and trunk rotation. A younger survivor would be more able to swivel his or her head to compensate for the loss of vision

• Have a brain that is more able to "absorb the impact" of the stroke. Younger adults have less age-related thinning of the cortex (the outer shell of the brain where brain rewiring occurs). Also, the blood vessels in the brain of young survivors tend to be healthier. All of these factors lead to a greater potential for brain rewiring.

- Are usually highly motivated. The bigger proportion of their life is yet to be lived. Their aspirations give them a huge advantage in their drive toward recovery.

- Can "bounce back" after injuries. For example, if a younger person has a fall, they can be expected to recover from any injuries faster and more completely.

In terms of recovery options, there are no differences in what helps recovery in the young and old, but the core concepts of stroke recovery can be expanded in YASS. Consider the word "**intensity**." That word is very popular in stroke rehab research. Intensity has to do with how much and how often a recovery option is used. Intensity is much like "dosage" in medication. The dosage has to do with how much and how often you take a medication. Generally, the more intensity (the higher the dosage), the better. YASS can do things that are more intensive because they have more energy.

Younger survivors have another advantage, as well: An easy acceptance of technology. Electrical stimulation, biofeedback, computer gaming, and so on, are technologies that can be very helpful at certain points in recovery. Younger stroke survivors may be more comfortable than older survivors with technologies that aid recovery.

Bottom line: What promotes recovery in both young and old is the same. However, younger survivors have more to put into recovery, and can expect more out of recovery. Age is one of the most important predictors of recovery after stroke. The closer you are to 25 years old, the better the recovery. More than 50 percent of young stroke survivors return to work. Young adult stroke survivors have much less of a chance to have a second stroke, as well. Approximately 33 percent of stroke survivors overall will have another stroke. In young adult survivors, the chance is much smaller—about 2 percent.

What Precautions Should Be Taken?

Many young stroke survivors are misdiagnosed when they first have their stroke. Many young people having a stroke are believed to be on illegal drugs. This is true even though the symptoms for stroke between the two groups (young and old) are similar. Part of this is because of the mistaken belief among medical professionals that stroke in young people is rare. However, while uncommon, stroke does happen in younger people. The misdiagnosis of stroke as a symptom of illegal drug use can delay time-sensitive treatment for younger survivors.

Young stroke survivors have more reason to modify risky behavior. Stopping smoking, for example, is more important to overall health to somebody who's 25 years old than somebody who's 95 years old.

While young survivors have more energy to put into recovery, the same precautions are just as important as with older survivors. Injuries hurt recovery. Always strive for recovery while also staying safe.

9 Recovery Machines

THOSE AMAZING MACHINES

Many researchers, medical doctors, and bioengineers dedicate much of their careers and cash to the development and marketing of stroke recovery machines. Why do they spend so much time and money on stroke recovery? Because there are 50 million stroke survivors worldwide, and it's a global economy. If an inventor brings one product to market and sells that product to just a small fraction of the 50 million, he stands to make a fortune. The tremendous potential for profit drives recovery machine development. This is promising news for stroke survivors. Many machines are already on the market, and more are on the way. It is wise for survivors to consider recovery machines now available, and keep an eye on emerging stroke-recovery technologies. It is also wise to keep an eye on people who make gizmos not to help but to profit from an often-vulnerable population.

Deciding which machines are appropriate for your recovery can be tricky. Much like picking and choosing other recovery options, picking machines is a matter of deciding what fits with!:

- Where you are in recovery
- What you need to accomplish
- How much you can afford
- What has independent evidence that it works

Stroke recovery technology can be expensive. On the other hand, some of these machines are designed to go home with you. This provides the opportunity for you to expand and magnify your at-home recovery effort without the ongoing aid of clinicians. In the long run, this can save time and money.

Many machines can help jump start a new phase in recovery. Other machines lessen the humdrum of **repetitive practice** by turning repetitive movements into a game. Some machines build muscle, some teach spastic muscles to relax, some encourage improved coordination, some help develop cardiovascular strength, and so forth. From walking to swallowing, and from visual deficits to speech impairments, there are machines that attempt to treat every movement deficit caused by stroke.

One other note: Many of the following machines use electrical stimulation (e-stim). Electrical stimulation after stroke is the single most important modality there is for recovery. Part of the reason e-stim is so important is that it does so many different things.

E-stim can be used in a variety of ways to help survivors. E-stim can . . .

- Start the neuroplastic process—e-stim changes the brain!
- Build muscle
- Stretch muscles
- Decrease the time between Botox is injected into muscles and the time muscles relax
- Increase the strength of the effect of Botox
- Start the neuroplastic process
- Fatigue spastic muscles so their antagonists (the muscles that work in the opposite direction) can work
- Increase tactile (touch) sensation
- Increase proprioception (the feeling of where the body is in space)

Work with your healthcare providers to incorporate e-stim into your recovery plan.

How Is It Done?

The following list provides broad categories of stroke recovery technologies. Included are general explanations of what machines in those categories do.

- *Cyclic electrical stimulation*: Cyclic electrical stimulation (**e-stim**) machines send electrical stimulation through electrodes to the skin overlying the muscles you want to work. This sort of e-stim may jump start movement in paralyzed muscles. It may also build bulk and strength in paralyzed muscles. Also, e-stim may relax muscles that are spastic by stimulating the muscles antagonistic (opposite) to the spastic muscles.

- *Electromyography (EMG)-based electrical stimulation (e-stim) with biofeedback*: These are e-stim machines with another feature added: The machine senses the effort of your muscles. If you tighten the muscle enough, you reach a threshold. Once you reach the threshold, the machine helps you complete the movement you are attempting. This process, called **biofeedback**, turns the passive activity provided by cyclic e-stim into an active exercise. Brain rewiring (**neuroplasticity**) is believed to occur because mental and/or physical effort is required.

- *E-stim orthotics*: These orthotics are worn on the recovering limbs. They differ from other forms of e-stim because they do not just "turn on and turn off" muscles. Instead, these orthotics stimulate muscles in the right way to do some real-world tasks. For instance, some e-stim orthotics lift the foot for people with **foot drop**. There are arm/hand orthotics that will help you open and close your hand, so you can grasp and release objects. These orthotics have the advantage of working on two levels:

  — They help you do some real-world tasks (e.g., grasping an object, walking). This **task-specific** training can promote recovery in that limb.

  — They encourage you to use the joints around the orthotic. For instance, an orthotic worn on the forearm and hand will also promote movement in the shoulder and elbow. In the leg, an orthotic that helps lift the foot will encourage improved movement from the hip and knee.

  — Unlike other forms of electrical stimulation, e-stim orthotics have the electrodes built in, eliminating or reducing the number of wires that tether the user to the machine.

- *Electromyography-based gaming*: These types of games work by sending information from muscles into a machine. These signals travel to the machine and guide a character or other game element on the screen. The machine uses your muscular effort to play a variety of video games, from solitaire to pinball.

- *Virtual reality (VR) gaming* (see the section You Are Game—Virtual Reality, in Chapter 4). There are now many virtual reality options for recovery from stroke. The two biggest are the Wii system by Nintendo and Microsoft's Xbox Kinect. The Wii allows you to move images on a TV screen by moving a hand-held controller. The Xbox Kinect is controller-free, using motion sensors that can track up to 48 points on your body to put you "in the game." Virtual reality gaming provides a safe, challenging, and fun environment in which to recover. Beyond the Wii and Xbox, many VR systems are inexpensive and plug directly into any TV with RCA type inputs. Therapists have even named this therapy: Wiihabilitation!

- *Bilateral arm trainers*: **Bilateral training** (BT) does not require equipment of any kind. For instance, walking is a form of BT. With every stride, the "good" leg provides guidance to the "bad" side about proper position and timing. There are machines that promote BT, however. Upper-extremity ergometers (stationary cycles used with arms or legs) are examples of simple bilateral trainers. Others include hand-crank upper-body ergometers, stationary bicycles, recumbent bilateral exercisers with arm components, and so forth.

- *Body weight-supported treadmill trainers*. A treadmill has many assets as a tool for relearning how to walk (see the section Train Well on a Treadmill in Chapter 2). One of the ways to safely use a treadmill, even for folks still unable to walk, is to support the weight of the body with a harness. These systems reduce the effect of gravity and also keep you safe if there is a loss of balance. Called **partial weight-supported treadmill (PWST) training**, this relatively low-tech safety apparatus is available at many rehabilitation hospitals. Some stroke survivors don't yet have the coordination to bring the "bad" leg forward while involved in PWSW. The assistance needed to move the leg forward can be provided by therapists crouched at the side of the treadmill. They literally grab the foot and leg and lift them off the ground to push them into the next step. The newer version of this technology has replaced therapists' hard work with a machine that moves the leg. An example of this sort of machine is the Lokomat®. Leg cuffs are attached to the hips, legs, ankles, and feet. The computer-driven leg cuffs progress the legs and feet in a way that promotes normal gait. This technology is quite expensive but is sometimes available at rehabilitation hospitals and other rehabilitation facilities. PWSW, when therapists assist leg movement, is much more low-tech. All that's needed is a treadmill and a harness. It can, however, be labor intensive if a therapist is needed to progress the foot during stepping.

- *Body weight-supported trainers without treadmills*: These trainers are weight support systems that allow you to carry less of your own weight as you relearn walking. A rolling platform suspends you while you walk on the floor. The amount of weight supported can be increased or decreased so, as you develop greater balance, the machine takes less of your weight. These machines include the NeuroGym® Bungee Walker, the Biodex Unweighing System, and the KineAssist™.

- *Cardiovascular machines*: Cardiovascular strength (stamina) directly impacts the amount and speed of recovery. Machines that increase stamina include treadmills, the NuStep®, and BioStep® **bilateral** trainer. Cardiovascular exercise is vital to recovery from stroke.

With any technology you use, consider the following:

- Ease of use
- Cost
- If it needs a therapist or doctor to implement
- If it can be used at home
- If there is a substantial amount of clinical research that shows positive results

Stroke-Recovery Machines and What They Do

A list of stroke-recovery machines with descriptions and contact information follows. *Note: The descriptions of these machines (in italics) were taken directly from the manufacturer and do not represent an endorsement by the author.*

Contact information can always be found on the website. The website will be the quickest, easiest, and maybe even the best source of information on these machines. If you, your doctor, or your treating therapist have any questions about acquiring and/or using the machine, the manufacturer is the best resource. Generally speaking, the manufacturer will know the most about:

- Cost
- If there are available lease options
- If you can buy used machines
- Insurance coverage (if any)

- Where to find the machine

- What research has been done on the machine

- If the machine is appropriate for your deficits

- Which therapists in your area are trained to use the machine

This section has three parts:

- Machine names and website(s) (if available) are listed.

- What the machine does, in the words of the manufacturer (in italics).

- The Status section tells if the machines are commercially available and if the stroke survivor can use them without help, or if supervision from a clinician is required.

Machines That Help Arm and Hand Movement and Function

- H200™ (www.bionessinc.com): *The H200 is a noninvasive device, worn on the forearm and hand that enables patients to perform everyday activities that were previously impossible. The NESS H200 can help the hand open and close, reduce stiffness, increase range of motion and strength, improve circulation, and assist in regaining awareness of an impaired limb. In addition to the amazing therapeutic benefits of the H200, patients have also embraced the comfort and ease of use of the system. Unlike other systems, the H200 orthosis incorporates a self-adjusting fit, to hold the wrist and hand in a functional position. This superior fit, coupled with the H200 electrode placement, allows patients to remove and replace the device without compromising therapy effectiveness. Also, the patented technology behind the H200 provides six different stimulation patterns to enable patients to perform a variety of tasks and use it for therapeutic activities, as well. The system is also versatile enough to be used in varied settings, including the home, with little technical expertise needed.*

  — STATUS: Commercially available. A therapist or physician should always supervise this treatment at the beginning. However, with training, this treatment can be done at home by the stroke survivor.

- MyoPro: *This is a portable, lightweight functional arm brace that restores movement to a weakened arm as a result of neuromuscular damage. The product incorporates a noninvasive myoelectric platform technology in a wearable device that enables a person to initiate and control his or her own motion. The portable arm brace has been proven effective in facilitating functional repetitive task practices during therapy and assist people in their daily living activities in the home. MyoPro technology does not use electrical impulses or stimulation. It reads weak muscle signals and sends them to the device's computer, which allows a person to move the affected arm.*

— STATUS: The Myomo MyoPro is a myoelectric limb orthosis available with a prescription from a Myomo-certified clinician. It may be reimbursed depending on medical necessity and the individual's insurance coverage.

- Armeo® (hocoma.com): *The Armeo facilitates intensive task-oriented upper extremity therapy after stroke, traumatic brain injury, or other neurological diseases and injuries. It combines an adjustable arm support, with augmented feedback and a large 3-D workspace that allows functional therapy exercises in a virtual reality environment.*

— STATUS: Not yet available in the United States.

- Hand Mentor™ (kineticmuscles.com): *The Hand Mentor™ is the first Active Repetitive Motion™ hand therapy device designed for use in therapy clinics to improve outcomes in stroke rehabilitation. The Hand Mentor™ actively involves the patient in his or her rehabilitation by encouraging self-initiated motion in the wrist and fingers, and assisting movement only when necessary.*

— STATUS: The "Pro" version, for treatment by therapists, is clinically available. The manufacturer is in the process of engineering an at-home version of the Hand Mentor™.

- SaeboFlex® (SaeboFlex.com): *The SaeboFlex™ positions the wrist and fingers into extension in preparation for functional activities. The user is able to grasp an object by voluntarily flexing his or her fingers. The extension spring system assists in re-opening the hand to release the object. Saebo equipment, especially the SaeboFlex™ orthosis, is specialized patented technology. Occupational and physical therapists attend specific education classes offered by Saebo, Inc. to become trained in the SaeboFlex®.*

— STATUS: Commercially available. A therapist or physician always supervises this treatment in the beginning. However, with training, there is potential for this treatment to be done by the stroke survivor, at home.

- Reo™ Go (motorika.com): *The Reo™ Go is a portable, easy-to-use system for delivering Reo Therapy. Combining streamlined ergonomic design and advanced software, the Reo™ Go provides a robust platform for highly effective robot-assisted upper extremity therapy.*

— STATUS: Commercially available. A therapist or physician should always supervise this treatment. This machine is expensive. However, treatment on this machine may not cost any more than typical physical-therapy treatments.

Machines That Help the Leg and Foot and Help Walking

- NESS L300™ (bionessinc.com): *The NESS L300™ utilizes proprietary technology that not only lets you walk smoother, but faster, as well. And, only the NESS L300™ has a built-in sensor that recognizes the surface you are walking on and adjusts accordingly. It is also a much more streamlined device compared to other available options. There are no bulky wires to deal with and the compact design even allows patients to wear their normal foot-wear. It's also easy for patients to use. Unlike some systems that can't easily be taken off and on, the NESS L300™ is surprisingly simple—making it ideal for inpatient or outpatient use.*

    — STATUS: Commercially available. A medical doctor or physical therapist supervises this treatment. However, the stroke survivor can also use this treatment at home during everyday walking.

- WalkAide (walkaide.com): *WalkAide uses advanced sensor technology to actually analyze the movement of your leg and foot. The system sends electrical signals to your peroneal nerve, which controls movement in your ankle and foot. These gentle electrical impulses activate the muscles to raise your foot at the appropriate time during the step cycle.*

    — STATUS: Commercially available. This treatment is supervised by a medical doctor or physical therapist. However, the stroke survivor can also use this treatment at home during everyday walking.

- LiteGait® (litegait.com): *LiteGait® is a therapy device used to promote the generation of normal walking patterns by controlling weight bearing, balance, and posture during walking therapy.*

    — STATUS: Commercially available. A therapist or physician always supervises this treatment.

- NeuroGym® Bungee Walker (neurogymtech.com): *The NeuroGym® Bungee Walker is a versatile body weight support mechanism enabling safe, intensive motor retraining. The unique patented design enables the re-training of gait and natural protective reactions by counteracting loss of stability as naturally as possible. Comparable to a pool environment in terms of support, the Bungee Walker allows graduated weight bearing while normal protective reactions such as sidestepping are re-developed.*

- STATUS: Commercially available. A therapist or physician always supervises this treatment in the beginning. However, with training, there is potential for this treatment to be done by the stroke survivor at home.

- **NxStep™** (biodex.com/rehab): *The Biodex NxStep Unweighing System enables partial weight-bearing therapy to be conducted with the assurance of patient comfort and safety, and with convenient access to the patient for manual assistance and observation.*

  - STATUS: Commercially available. A therapist or physician always supervises this treatment in the beginning. However, with training, there is potential for this treatment to be done by the stroke survivor at home.

- Gait Trainer 3™ (biodex.com/rehab): *The Gait Trainer 3™ has an instrumented deck that monitors and records step length, step speed, and right-to-left time distribution (step symmetry). Patients are motivated by the real-time audio and visual biofeedback. They are prompted into proper gait patterns, step length, step speed, and step symmetry.*

  - STATUS: Commercially available. A therapist or physician always supervises this treatment in the beginning. However, with training, there is potential for this treatment to be done by the stroke survivor at home.

- Lokomat® (hocoma.com/products/lokomat): *Locomotion therapy supported by an automated gait orthosis on a treadmill has established itself as an effective intervention for improving over-ground walking function caused by neurological diseases and injuries. The Lokomat is the first driven gait orthosis that assists walking movements of gait-impaired patients and is used to improve mobility in individuals following stroke, spinal cord injury, traumatic brain injury, multiple sclerosis, or other neurological diseases and injuries.*

  - STATUS: Commercially available. A therapist or physician always supervises this treatment. This machine is very expensive. However, treatment on this machine may not cost any more than typical physical therapy treatments.

- Reo Ambulator (motorika.com): *Reo Ambulator is an innovative robotic gait training device that integrates body weight support treadmill training (BWSTT) with advanced robotics to help rehabilitate patients who experience neuromuscular dysfunction to address problems with ambulation, balance, coordination, posture, and stamina.*

— STATUS: Commercially available. A therapist or physician always supervises this treatment. This machine is very expensive. However, treatment on this machine may not cost any more than typical physical therapy treatments.

- KineAssist™ (kineadesign.com): *KineAssist™ technology will allow therapists to safely challenge patients in functional environments with reduced concern about falls, record objective measures, and integrate with existing practice settings.*

  — STATUS: Commercially available. A therapist or physician always supervises this treatment.

Machines That Can Be Used for the Upper or Lower Extremities

- NeuroMove™ (neuromove.com): *The NeuroMove™ works by detecting the attempts to move a muscle group sent from the brain. These attempts are shown in the display as significant increases in the signal over regular muscle activity. The built-in microprocessor intelligently distinguishes between regular muscle activity, muscle tone, noise, and real attempts. When a real attempt is detected, the unit "rewards" the patient with a few seconds of muscle contraction, where the visual and sensory feedback serve as an important element in relearning the movement.*

  — STATUS: Commercially available. A therapist or physician always supervises this treatment in the beginning. However, with training, there is potential for this treatment to be done by the stroke survivor at home.

- Biomove 3000 (biomove.com/biomove-home): *The system is able to detect the extremely small electrical EMG signals still measurable in paralyzed muscles after a stroke. These tiny signals are used to initiate an electrical stimulation impulse to the same muscles, resulting in actual muscle movement!*

  — STATUS: Commercially available. A therapist or physician always supervises this treatment in the beginning. However, with training, there is potential for this treatment to be done by the stroke survivor at home.

- Interactive Metronome (IM) and Gait Mate (interactivemetronome .com): *The Interactive Metronome is an advanced brain-based treatment program designed to promote and enhance brain performance and recovery. This is accomplished by using innovative neurosensory and neuromotor exercises.*

IM also makes the Gait Mate, which is described like this: The therapist inserts a wireless insole into the patient's shoe that detects when the patient performs a heel strike. The patient hears a beat through wireless headphones or speakers and is asked to match the cadence provided. The Gait Mate provides the patient with auditory feedback as he or she walks, with instruction to speed up if walking too slowly or to slow down if shuffling or dropping his or her foot too quickly. The patient receives no positive feedback if his or her heel doesn't strike the ground.

— STATUS: Commercially available. A therapist or physician always supervises this treatment in the beginning. However, with training, there is potential for this treatment to be done by the stroke survivor at home.

Machines for Other Aspects of Stroke Recovery

- VitalStim Therapy (vitalstimtherapy.com): *VitalStim Therapy uses small electrical currents to stimulate the muscles responsible for swallowing. At the same time, trained specialists help patients "re-educate" their muscles through rehabilitation therapy.*

  — STATUS: Commercially available. A therapist or physician always supervises this treatment.

- NovaVision VRT™ Vision Restoration Therapy™ (novavision.com): *VRT is a clinically proven, FDA-cleared technology designed to improve the quality of life of stroke and brain injury patients by restoring some of their lost vision. The therapy does not require surgery or medication of any kind.*

  — STATUS: Commercially available. A therapist or physician always supervises this treatment. This machine is expensive. However, treatment on this machine may not cost any more than typical physical therapy treatments.

- This list of machines is not complete, nor can it be. The rapid development of these new technologies means that new products become available every day.

Future Machines

The best way to stay abreast of the latest and greatest recovery machines is to "keep your ear to the ground." Check the Internet, TV, and print for new ideas. The best outlet for information on cutting-edge machines for stroke rehabilitation is a website called Medgadget (medgadget.com/rehab). The free magazines, *Stroke Smart* (strokesmart.org) and *Stroke Connection* (strokeassociation.org), have great suggestions for new machines. The advertisements in these magazines provide a wealth of information, photographs, and contact information on commercially available stroke recovery machines. There are also articles that review the latest stroke recovery technology.

As time goes on, stroke recovery will rely more and more on machines. The most difficult part of this new machine-driven world of recovery is figuring out how to use these machines. Using some machines is as simple as placing a couple of electrodes and flipping a switch. Other machines are so complex that without a highly trained person, the machine is virtually useless. Some rehabilitation hospitals spend tens of thousands of dollars on machines that end up collecting dust. If the machine takes too long to learn, therapists won't use it. Also, if setting up the machine for a patient to use takes too long, then the machine will not be used. My hope, as we move forward, is that the folks who make these machines understand that simplicity of use is essential. If a machine is simple and effective, survivors will be inclined to buy it and use it at home. Or, if a therapist is needed, the machine needs to be simple enough to not burn available treatment time with a protracted set-up.

What Precautions Should Be Taken?

Make sure your doctor knows if you decide to add a machine to your recovery efforts. Some machines require a doctor's prescription. Contact individual manufacturers to determine if the machine needs a doctor's prescription. These machines may or may not be covered by insurance, depending on a number of factors. Again, the manufacturers will know if their machine is covered. They are in business to serve you, so you will find them helpful and informative as you consider their machine.

Recovery options that involve electrical stimulation have precautions and contraindications. Discuss these with your medical doctor prior to using any electrical stimulation options. Here is a partial list of contraindications and precautions for recovery options that use electrical stimulation:

- Pregnancy
- Skin irritation
- Epilepsy/seizures

- Sensitive skin
- Compromised sensation
- Heart disease
- Pacemakers or defibrillators
- Recent surgery if muscle contraction may disrupt healing
- Electrode placement over the carotid sinus in the neck
- Existing thrombosis

Resources

WEBSITES

The Stronger After Stroke blog

Website address: recoverfromstroke.blogspot.com

The Stronger After Stroke blog is the companion website to this book. The latest stroke recovery information is available with commentary, embedded links, and video. There are also clickable links to a ton of resources. Included are stroke-specific resources on drug warnings, finances, insurance coverage, nationwide stroke center, stroke support group searches, and more.

The Evidence-Based Review of Stroke Rehabilitation (EBRSR)

Website address: www.ebrsr.com

The EBRSR is an easy way of accessing the latest and greatest that stroke-rehabilitation research has to offer. Each section (called a module) opens with an easy-to-read list that explains which therapies work, which do not, and which are promising but still unproven. Not only that, but it is updated every six months.

The Evidence-Based Review of Moderate to Severe Acquired Brain Injury (ABIEBR)

Website address: www.abiebr.com

The ABIEBR provides information about brain injury and how to recover from it. The information in this website is easy to access and easy-to-understand. Although the website is about brain injury, much of its information is directly applicable to stroke and stroke recovery.

The StrokEngine

Website address: www.strokengine.ca

From acupuncture to virtual reality, the StrokEngine is called "the stroke rehabilitation intervention website." StrokEngine allows you to look up individual therapies to see if they hold promise for you. Once you've chosen a therapy, go to the section called Patient/Family Info. Once there, go to the section called Does It Work for Stroke? This section gets to the bottom line about that particular therapy.

Medgadget

Website address: www.medgadget.com/rehab

This website reviews the latest technology (machines) for stroke recovery.

PUBLICATIONS

Stroke Connection (Published by the American Stroke Association)

Subscription Information:
Call: 1-888-478-7653.
E-mail: strokeconnection@heart.org
Website address: www.strokeassociation.org
Cost: Free

Stroke Smart (Published by the National Stroke Association)

Subscription Information
Call: 1-800-787-6537
Website address: www.strokesmart.org
Cost: Free

CLINICAL TRIALS

If you are interested in getting therapy beyond what your insurance will provide, consider involvement in stroke-recovery research. Research trials often offer treatment options that are not available in any other clinical setting. There are research trials happening all over the country. Here are three Internet sites that have lists of ongoing trials.

Run by the National Institute of Health

Website address: www.clinicaltrials.gov

Run by the Internet Stroke Center at Washington University School of Medicine:

Website address: www.strokecenter.org/trials

Run by Centerwatch, a Business of Jobson Medical Information

Website address: www.centerwatch.com

Glossary

Active movement

Movement done with the stroke survivor's own muscle power.

Active range of motion (AROM)

The arc of movement of a joint that the stroke survivor can perform with his or her own power.

Acute phase

Broadly, the first seven days after stroke. After the acute phase is the **subacute phase**.

Adaptive equipment

Any equipment that makes the life of stroke survivors easier or gives them the ability to do a task that they would not otherwise be able to do. This term tends to be used interchangeably with **assistive devices**.

AFO

See ankle-foot orthoses.

Ankle-foot orthoses (AFO)

An orthotic designed to lift the foot and stabilize the ankle during walking.

Aphasia

A general term for the inability to either speak (expressive aphasia) or understand speech (receptive aphasia). Aphasia affects approximately 20 percent of survivors who have had a left-sided stroke (right side of the body affected). Used interchangeably with the word *dysphasia*.

Apraxic (apraxia)

Survivors with apraxia have two problems: They (1) cannot tell where their limb is in space without looking at it and (2) have an inability to plan movements. Apraxia makes quality movement difficult or impossible, even when survivors have enough active range of motion and strength.

Assistive devices

Any equipment that makes the life of stroke survivors easier or gives them the ability to do a task that they would not otherwise be able to do. This term tends to be used interchangeably with the term **adaptive equipment**.

Balance training

Any recovery technique used to increase balance after stroke. Traditionally, balance training is done in a rehabilitation facility by a physical therapist.

Bilateral

Using either both of the upper or both of the lower extremities at the same time.

Bilateral training

Any recovery technique that involves repetitive and predictable patterned movement of either both of the upper extremities, or both of the lower extremities at the same time. Bilateral training falls into two main categories: (1) equal and at the same time (as in conducting an orchestra) and (2) equal and alternating (as in drumming using alternating hands).

Biofeedback

A system that allows for continuous monitoring of a body system in order to control that body system. Biofeedback happens all over the body all the time. For instance, in a simple biofeedback loop, to relax a muscle, you send signals to the muscle to contract and the muscle sends back a signal that tells you that the muscle is relaxed. Biofeedback is traditionally used to allow for control over systems in the body that are not normally controllable, like heart rate and blood pressure. In stroke survivors who want to move better, biofeedback can be used to monitor the contraction of a muscle or group of muscles that are not responding in order to encourage muscle contraction. An example of biofeedback used in stroke recovery is electromyography-based biofeedback machines.

Brain derived neurotrophic factor (BDNF)

Neuroscientists refer to be BDNF as "Miracle Grow™ for the brain." BDNF is naturally produced by the brain after brain injury, including stroke. BDNF is an essential ingredient to driving the necessary neuroplastic change for motor recovery (relearning of movement) after stroke. BDNF helps neurons (nerve cells) in the brain form (synaptic) connections. A small percentage of survivors do not produce BDNF after their stroke. There is a genetic test to determine if a particular survivor produces BDNF. If the survivor does not produce BDNF, clinical decisions about rehabilitation can be based on that information.

Brunnström, Signe

Signe Brunnström, a Swedish Fulbright scholar and pioneer physical therapist was the first to map out the predictable **stages of recovery** from stroke. Although Hippocrates described stroke some 2,400 years earlier, Brunnström was the first to describe the landmarks on the road to recovery. These predictable stages of recovery are commonly called "Brunnström's stages of recovery." Some of the tests that Brunnström developed decades ago are still used in rehabilitation research, and the results of those tests tend to correlate well with more sophisticated computer-driven tests like testing of neuroplasticity by functional magnetic resonance imaging (fMRI) and transcranial magnetic stimulation (TMS).

Brunnström's stages of recovery

The six predictable stages that stroke survivors experience during recovery from stroke. These stages go from Stage 1, in which the stroke survivor is flaccid, to Stage 6, in which the stroke survivor is fully recovered.

Cardiovascular

Having to do with the heart and blood vessels. The term *cardiovascular* tends to be used to describe endurance of the heart and lungs.

Cardiovascular training

Training focused on increasing endurance of the heart and lungs.

Central obesity

Described as apple-shaped, a body shape where the waist is larger than the hips. This shape, as opposed to carrying weight around the hips, has been shown to have increased risk of high blood pressure, diabetes, heart disease, and stroke.

Chronic phase

The term used to describe a stroke survivor's time since stroke. The chronic phase after stroke is usually considered to be the period that is more than three months to a year after stroke. The harkening of the chronic phase is the **plateau**; once the survivor's recovery plateaus, that survivor is said to be in the chronic phase. The chronic phase continues to the end of life. Before the chronic phase is the **subacute** phase. The **subacute** phase is usually considered to be the period from seven days to three months after stroke.

Complex regional pain syndrome (CRPS)

In stroke, CRPS is often in the arm and hand and is triggered by the trauma inflicted on the shoulder joint by the stroke. In this case, CRPS it is typically called *shoulder-hand syndrome* (SHS). Up to 25 percent of all stroke survivors get SHS. Symptoms of SHS include pain; swelling; stiffness;

considerable reduction of movement in shoulder joint, wrist, and hand; discoloration of the skin.

SHS usually starts one to six months after stroke. Pain usually starts in the shoulder and moves down the arm to the hand. SHS tends to get worse over time and can make movement very painful. The pain limits the amount and type of movement the survivor is willing to do, which can affect recovery. If left untreated, SHS can result in deformity and "frozen shoulder" (the tissue around the shoulder becomes stiff and movement at the shoulder becomes painful).

Research suggests SHS is caused by the changes in how the shoulder moves after stroke. Poor quality of movement of the shoulder causes microscopic injury to the shoulder joint. The injury to the shoulder effects the nervous system. The nervous system reacts to the injury by sending intense pain signals to the arm and hand. Treatments include: passive range of motion exercises; corticosteroids (steroids); NSAIDs (aspirin, ibuprofen, naproxen sodium, etc.); centrally acting analgesics; and physical and occupational therapy.

Compensatory movement, compensation
Relying on the unaffected limbs to do the activities of daily living.

Component parts (of a task), practice of
Also known as **part-whole practice**, individual movements that, when put together, form the movements needed to do a **task**. This concept is used in constraint-induced therapy. The entire task is broken down to component parts. The component (individual) parts (movements) are practiced individually. Once those components parts are individually mastered, they are put together to do the entire task. The thinking is, if a survivor attempts to do the whole task it will be "overwhelming to the nervous system," and the survivor will get frustrated and fail. But if the complex task is broken down to its component parts, the parts are easier to learn.

Constraint-induced therapy (CIT) for the arm
Traditional CIT is a stroke-recovery technique that involves constraining the "good" arm and hand and having the stroke survivor only use the affected arm and hand in a clinical setting.

Constraint-induced therapy for the leg (leg CIT)
Four different schools of thought debate the exact definition of leg CIT: providing extensive and intensive exercises of the affected leg; partial weight-supported walking; electrical stimulation ankle-foot orthoses; or

providing a shoe lift or some other type of orthotic on the unaffected side, forcing weight onto the affected side.

Contracture

A shortening of soft tissue (e.g., muscle, nerves, blood vessels). A contracture happens when a joint is left flexed for too long and the soft tissue shortens. In stroke survivors, contracture may occur in response to spastic muscles, which are in a constant state of contraction.

Conventional therapy

The usual care offered in a particular setting. After stroke, survivors are usually offered conventional therapy, which consists of standard occupational, physical, and speech therapies.

Comorbidity (comorbidities)

Besides the stroke, all the other illnesses (including behavioral or mental) and/or injuries the survivor has. Examples include diabetes, hip pain, and chronic headaches. Comorbidities can have a profound impact on recovery.

Core

The portion of the brain killed by the stroke. Contrast with penumbra.

Discharged

Released from therapy. "Discharged" is the technical term that therapists use to describe the point at which therapy is ended. Different therapeutic disciplines (e.g., physical, occupational, speech therapies) may end at different times, depending on the progression, or lack of progression, of the stroke survivor. Therapists will usually continue therapy until they perceive that progress toward recovery has ended. Therapists call this lack of progress a **plateau**. The point at which any patient is discharged for any therapy is also dictated by the strict parameters set up by insurance companies, both private and governmental.

Distributed practice

A schedule of practice in which learning a new movement or skill is spread out over time. Distributed practice schedules are typically used in rehabilitation facilities. For instance, a typical rehabilitation schedule might be three sessions per week, 45 minutes each session, or five sessions a week for one hour. Contrast with **massed practice**.

Dorsal root rhizotomy (selective dorsal rhizotomy)

Neurosurgery that selectively destroys nerve roots (parts of the nerve) in the spinal cord and leads to a reduction or elimination of spasticity. It is most often used in children with spastic cerebral palsy. However, it is also effective in adults with profound spasticity after stroke. It is not reversible (once the nerve roots are cut you cannot put them back together again). Also, dorsal root rhizotomy (DRR) eliminates sensation because it destroys the nerve roots that transmit sensation from the muscle to the spinal cord. It should be considered in survivors with profound spasticity that is painful and risks injury to skin (pressure sores).

Dorsiflexion

The movement of the foot upward when only the ankle joint is moved. If you are sitting in a chair with your feet on the ground and you want to tap your foot, the first movement of the foot, upward, is dorsiflexion. In many stroke survivors, this movement is limited or lost. The verb is "dorsiflex." A lack of ability to dorsiflex is called **drop foot** or **foot drop**.

Drop foot or foot drop

A reduced or eliminated ability to lift (dorsiflex) the foot at the ankle. The result of drop foot is *toe dragging*.

Dysarthria

Weakness or paralysis of the muscles of the mouth that form words. Dysarthria refers to impairments in speech caused by a reduced ability to use the muscles associated with speech. Dysarthria may affect the muscles of the mouth, lips, tongue, face, and respiratory system. Dysarthria is caused by damage, from the stroke, to the part of the brain that controls the movement of the mouth. Dysarthria can be reduced by the same mechanisms that reduce disability in the limbs, including **repetitive practice**. Contrast with **expressive aphasia**.

Electrical stimulation

See neuromuscular electrical stimulation.

Electrical stimulation ankle-foot orthosis (or "orthotics")

A group of commercially available orthotics designed to use electrical stimulation to lift the foot (**dorsiflexion**) in people with drop foot.

Electromyography (EMG)

The testing of muscles as they contract (flex) and relax. Electromyography is often used to evaluate spastic muscles. It is also used in some electrical stimulation stroke-recovery machines to provide feedback to the machine regarding the amount of muscular effort by the stroke survivor.

Electromyography (EMG)-based electrical stimulation

Electrical stimulation that "rewards" the stroke survivor who tries to move a limb that is (or is nearly) immobile. If the stroke survivor tries to move the limb, electrical stimulation is sent to the muscles that complete the desired movement. Some of these machines are quite sensitive and can detect a signal even when no movement is visually apparent. Machines in this class include Mentamove, the Biomove 3000 system, and NeuroMove™.

Embolitic stroke

A stroke caused by an embolism (usually a blood clot) that travels from another part of the body and lodges in and clogs an artery leading to the brain or in the brain. The embolism cuts off the blood supply to part of the brain, causing stroke.

E-stim

Electrical stimulation. *See* neuromuscular electrical stimulation.

Evidence-based practice

Basing treatment of a patient on the best available research, as well as sound clinical judgment. It is of considerable benefit for stroke survivors to make sure that the treatment techniques they are using, with or without administration by a therapist, are evidence based.

Expressive aphasia

The loss or limitation of communicating, either through the spoken word or the written one. Expressive aphasia is caused by damage to the language centers of the brain. Stroke survivors sometimes have expressive aphasia if they have had a left-sided stroke (right side of the body affected).

FES

See functional electrical stimulation.

Foot drop

An inability to **dorsiflex** (lift the foot at the ankle).

Forced use

Having the survivor constrain the "good" arm/hand using a sling and/or mitt for most of their waking hours. Forced use is different from constraint-induced therapy (CIT). CIT involves forced use. CIT also involves supervised task practice. Forced use does not involve supervised task practice.

Functional

A term used by insurance companies and therapists to describe the ability to do a real-world task. For instance, if stroke survivors are able to dress themselves, no matter how they do it, they are said to be functional in dressing. The word "functional" does not address the deficits of the affected ("bad") side of the stroke survivor.

Functional electrical stimulation

Low levels of electrical stimulation run from a machine, through wires, and into electrodes put on the surface of the skin overlying the muscles involved in a functional task. The electricity contracts the muscles in a precise pattern that allows for a specific task to be accomplished.

Greater trochanter

A large bump that is at the top of the femur (the large bone that forms the top half of the leg). This bump is the surface that often hits the ground first when someone with a stroke falls. Discreet hip pads that can be worn inside undergarments will protect the vulnerable part of the hip during a fall.

Hemiparesis

Half the body is partially paralyzed. Hemiparesis is often incorrectly used to describe **hemiplegia**.

Hemiplegia

Total paralysis of the head, arm, leg, and trunk on one side of the body, whereas **hemiparesis** is weakness on one side of the body. Hemiplegia is often incorrectly used to describe hemiparesis.

Hemorrhagic stroke

A stroke in which a blood vessel bursts and blood is released into the brain. Hemorrhagic strokes make up approximately 20 percent of all strokes. The classic question to determine the type of stroke that a stroke survivor had is, "Was your stroke a bleed (hemorrhagic) or a block (**ischemic**)?"

Home Exercise Program (HEP)

Traditionally, therapists have viewed the home exercise program (HEP) as a series of exercises that followed two rules: (1) The exercises given to the stroke survivor right before the therapist discharged the survivor, and (2) the exercises were the same exercises that the stroke survivor had done with the therapist in the clinic. These are the same exercises that have precipitated the plateau that caused the survivor to be discharged. If done correctly, a HEP can provide two important ingredients to the process of recovery: (1) A robust HEP can allow the survivor to continue to recover even after they've been discharged from therapy, and (2) while in therapy with the therapists, a HEP can expand the amount of practice time per day. In this way, the HEP expands the therapeutic experience the same way a child's homework expands the time allotted to learning a subject.

Hyperacute phase

The hyperacute phase is broadly from the first symptom through the first six hours after stroke. This phase is "hyper" important because "Time is brain." That is, the faster the survivor can get to the hospital, the more brain can be saved. This phase includes the only period of time in which strong clot-busting medications (like tissue plasminogen activator, or TPA) can be administered. Immediately following the hyperacute phase is the **acute phase**.

Imagery

See mental practice.

Intensity

In exercise physiology, intensity refers to the frequency and duration of training as well as the amount of energy expended when exercising. With regard to stroke rehabilitation, intensity has shown to positively affect recovery. Human and animal studies indicate that increased intensity nets increased changes in cortical reorganization (brain plasticity).

Ischemic stroke

A stroke in which blood is blocked from going through an artery that leads to or resides in the brain. The way the artery is blocked further distinguishes between two separate types of ischemic strokes: (1) **thrombotic stroke** and (2) **embolic stroke**.

Learned nonuse

The result of trying and failing a movement so often that the stroke survivor believes that the effort is futile. With lack of attempt comes shrinkage of the part of the brain that was used for that movement prior to the stroke. Researchers believe that survivors can overcome learned nonuse with interventions that force use, such as **constraint-induced therapy**.

Mass synergies

A large set of movements where no single movement can be done alone. In stroke survivors, during some periods in the arc of recovery, movements cannot be isolated. That is, stroke survivors cannot just do one (e.g., reaching forward) without doing a whole series of movements (e.g., the upper arm coming away from the body, the elbow bending). All the movements, when taken together, define mass synergies. *See also* **synergistic movement** and **synergy**.

Massed practice

A schedule of practice in which learning a new movement or skill is done many hours a day, usually over a two- to three-week period. Massed practice schedules are not typically used in rehabilitation facilities. However, **constraint-induced therapy** (CIT) is usually done using a massed-practice schedule. CIT has traditionally used a schedule of five to eight hours per day, for two to three weeks. Contrast with **distributed practice**.

Melodic intonation therapy (MIT)

A speech therapy that uses simple and exaggerated melodic elements to recreate speech. Because the area of the brain that typically processes music is on the opposite side of the brain that typically processes language, MIT aims to use undamaged parts of the brain to compensate for the language areas of the brain affected by stroke.

Mental practice

A technique long used by athletes and musicians to precisely imagine physical movements in an attempt to enhance performance during the actual event. Traditionally known as "imagery," mental practice consists of deep relaxation followed by a disciplined practice of imagining moving the same way as prior to the stroke. Research indicates that mental practice may increase quality of movement in stroke survivors.

Meta-analysis

Essentially, a "study of studies" where all the available studies of a subject are evaluated based on a set of pre-established criteria. Once the studies are evaluated, they are given a certain weight and run through a mathematical formula. A meta-analysis dedicated to stroke recovery gives scores to all the recovery strategies for which there is available research and distinguishes "winners" from "lemons." The definitive stroke recovery meta-analysis is the Evidence-based Review of Stroke Rehabilitation by Dr. Robert Teasell and colleagues at the University of Western Ontario, Canada. This amazing stroke-specific document can be found on the web at www.ebrsr.com.

Mirror therapy

A therapy in which the stroke survivor copies the movement of the "good" upper extremity with the "bad" extremity while looking at the unaffected side via a mirror. The mirror gives the optical illusion that the affected extremity is moving perfectly. This therapy is thought to provide the brain with fake, but normalizing, information, fooling the brain into rewiring in a way that allows for more normal movement.

Modified constraint-induced therapy (mCIT)

A form of **constraint-induced therapy** that uses a schedule that is available within the normal schedule of typical outpatient settings. Developed by noted stroke researcher Dr. Stephen J. Page (with the help of the author of this book), mCIT involves the stroke survivor seeing a therapist three times a week for half-hour sessions. At home, the stroke survivor constrains the affected arm for five hours during a time when he or she is wakeful and active. Many rehabilitation facilities have modified mCIT even further in order to reflect the particular skills of their therapists and to reflect the particular resources available at their facilities.

Motor learning

A form of learning that involves the cognitive endeavor of learning new movements. For survivors, motor learning is a combination of motor learning and motor relearning. Motor learning involves establishing new brain pathways, while motor relearning involves re-establishing brain pathways that existed prior to the stroke.

Necessity drives recovery

A phrase that describes the fact that *needing* to do a valued, real-world task (necessity) promotes recovery. The more essential a task is to a survivor, the more the task can be used to focus efforts toward accomplishment of the task.

Neuro

A prefix that means "nerve." *Neuro* is used as a prefix for anything that has to do with nerves, as in neurorecovery or **neuroplasticity**. Stroke is damage to the nerves of the brain.

Neuromuscular electrical stimulation (NMES)

The sort of electrical stimulation that causes muscles to contract. A machine delivers specific amounts of electrical stimulation down a wire and into an electrode that, with the use of a sticky gel, attaches to the skin overlying the muscles that are to be stimulated. Even muscles that are paralyzed after stroke respond to NMES. This treatment has shown promise as a way of retaining range of motion, muscle strength, and may even help jump start movement in **paretic** limbs. Neuromuscular electrical stimulation can be used in the arm or leg. Many companies are developing machines that provide NMES in orthotics, which allow the stroke survivor to move and practice everyday tasks, often with independence from tethering wires.

Neuroplasticity, neuroplastic, neuroplastically

The ability for neurons (nerve cells) to communicate with each other in new and ever-changing ways. Research using brain-imaging techniques has shown that neuroplasticity allows stroke survivors to recover by rearranging neuronal connections to "go around" the area of the brain damaged by stroke. It has been demonstrated that with the correct type, intensity, and schedule of practice, neuroplasticity can reallocate a part of the brain to any task practiced.

Paralysis

The complete loss of muscle control.

Paresis, paretic
Partial loss of muscle control. The adjective is *paretic*.

Partial weight-supported treadmill training
The stroke survivor wears a harness attached to risers that are then attached to a suspension device so that the stroke survivor can be suspended over a treadmill on which he or she walks.

Part-whole practice
See **Component parts (of a task), practice of**

Partial weight-supported walking (PWSW)
Walking while part of the weight of the stroke survivor is reduced, which lessens the effect of gravity and protects the stroke survivor if balance is lost. The reduction of body weight can be accomplished in two ways: (1) Having the stroke survivor wear a harness that is attached to risers. The risers are attached to a suspension device so that the stroke survivor can be suspended over a treadmill. (2) Having the stroke survivor supported through the pelvis in a mobile wheeled device. Once the stroke survivor is secure in the device, the device provides adequate lift to allow walking over ground. The KineAssist™ and NeuroGym® Bungee Walker are examples of this technology.

Passive movement
Movement that is not performed by the person's own muscular power. For example, passive movement of the elbow would involve someone besides the stroke survivor moving the joint. However, passive movement can be done by the stroke survivor himself or herself, as well. For instance, if the stroke survivor moves the affected elbow with the unaffected hand, then the "bad" elbow is said to be involved in passive movement. Passive movement of the affected limbs is often an important part of reducing the risk of contracture and retaining **passive range of motion**. Some research indicates that passive movement may drive positive neuroplastic change.

Passive range of motion (PROM)
The amount of movement available in a joint when the joint is moved with **passive movement**. For example, the PROM of the elbow would be the amount of movement measured from the angle of the most flexion (elbow bent) to the angle of the elbow when it is most extended (elbow straight).

Patient driven

The term used to describe two separate ideas: (1) **Neuroplasticity** in the brain is "driven" by the stroke survivor. Stroke survivors "drive" their own nervous systems during voluntary effort, and through this process, neuroplastic changes in the brain occur. (2) Therapies are said to be "patient driven" when, with little training and/or set up, the patient can do the therapies by himself or herself.

Peer-reviewed

The term used for research articles that have been scrutinized by experts in the field. For instance, an article about a new treatment for the recovery from stroke might be published in a peer-reviewed journal. If so, this article has a high chance of being accurate and reliable. However, much of what is published, either in books, newspapers, and magazines and on the Internet, does not go through the peer-review process and, therefore, is not considered as reliable as peer-reviewed information. If the source is simply reporting what a peer-reviewed article said, then it may be a reliable resource. Keep in mind that the mainstream media may misinterpret what was originally published in a peer-reviewed article. In any case, when researching different ways of recovering from stroke, look for information that was originally published in journals that are peer-reviewed.

Penumbra

The area next to the part of the brain killed by the stroke. The penumbra contain cells that are "stunned"—not dead, but not functioning. In the **subacute phase** after stroke, the penumbra begins to resolve, and as it does, recovery is often rapid. The penumbra is an area of the brain that can either be useful (be used much of the same way it was prior to the stroke) or be useless (be used very little after stroke). The process of rendering the penumbra as useless is known as learned nonuse.

Percutaneous

A medical procedure, where the skin is punctured to access tissue under the skin.

Percutaneous NMES (perc-NMES)

A form of **neuromuscular electrical stimulation** where the stimulation is delivered under the skin to the muscles. For instance, percutaneous electrical stimulation is sometimes used to reduce shoulder **subluxation** (shoulder dislocation) after stroke.

Physiatrist
A medical doctor specifically trained in physical medicine and rehabilitation. Often called "stroke doctors" by stroke survivors, these doctors have special medications, measurements, and treatments to help stroke survivors recover.

Plateau, plateaued
A word that means "flattening out," used to describe the point at which a stroke survivor is no longer making progress. Different therapeutic interventions (e.g., physical, occupational, and speech therapy) may plateau at different times. A plateau in progress may be more reflective of ineffective treatment options, ineffective implementations of treatment options, or incorrect dosages, rather than an actual halting of potential.

Proprioception
The feeling of where parts of the body (e.g., arms and legs) are in space without actually looking at the specific body part. The information about where the body is in space is delivered to the brain from little organs in the muscle and tendons called proprioceptors.

Range of motion (ROM)
The largest arc of movement of a joint. Range of motion is broken down into two categories: **active range of motion (AROM)** and **passive range of motion (PROM)**.

Receptive aphasia
An inability to understand spoken language. Stroke survivors sometimes have receptive aphasia when they have had a left-sided stroke (right side of the body affected).

Reciprocal innervation
A phenomenon first described by Nobel laureate Sir Charles Sherrington that describes the fact that for a muscle (agonist) to contract, the muscle that opposes that muscle (antagonist) has to relax. For instance, in order for the muscles that bend the elbow to work, the muscles that straighten the elbow must "agree" to relax. This intricate dance between muscles is controlled subconsciously by the spinal cord, not the brain.

Repetitive practice
Repeating a movement or series of movements in order to drive neuroplastic change to benefit future attempts at the same movement.

Resistance training

Any training in which muscles work against an opposing force. The most common type of resistance training is weightlifting. This sort of exercise is essential to recovery from stroke.

Resolution of the penumbra

A reduction of swelling in the brain that leads to rapid recovery in the few weeks to months after the stroke. The **penumbra,** the area in which swelling is reduced, is next to the nerve cells in the brain killed by the stroke.

Rhythmic auditory cuing

Using a steady beat generated by a metronome, drum machine, or music to establish a tempo that the stroke survivor tries to match by doing a particular movement or set of movements on the sound of the beat.

Rhythmicity, Rhythmic

The inherent rhythm in something. In recovery from stroke, rhythm can be used to motivate and provide an auditory cue. For instance, having one hand reach out and hit a target may help the stroke survivor learn to move, but if the same exercise is done while trying to hit the target on the snare beat for an entire song, then the exercise becomes motivating and more challenging.

Serial casting

A proven method for increasing the length of muscles shortened by spasticity and/or weakness. During serial casting, a cast is placed around a joint in a lengthened position so that the muscle is gradually and continually stretched.

Sherrington, Sir Charles

The scientist who, in the late 1800s and early 1900s, developed the foundation of modern physical and occupational therapy. In addition to a huge amount of neurological discoveries and observations, Nobel Prize winner Sherrington described **reciprocal innervation** and **proprioception,** two essential concepts in the recovery from stroke.

Shoulder-hand syndrome (SHS)

See complex regional pain syndrome (CRPS)

Soft tissue

The "meat" of the body that surrounds organs and bones. Included are muscles, tendons, ligaments, fat, fascia, nerve fibers, blood vessels, and joint tissue. In stroke survivors, soft tissue has the potential to irreversibly shorten because the affected joints are held in flexed postures. A comprehensive stretching program is essential to keeping soft tissue long enough so that, if and when control over the joints is re-established, there is enough soft tissue length to accommodate the "new" movement. If soft tissue is not stretched enough, an irreversible shortening of soft tissue, called a **contracture,** can develop.

Spasticity, spastic

Tight and sometimes locked muscles caused by impulses from the spinal cord. The part of the brain that normally communicates with the muscles dies during the stroke. The muscles need protection from being torn, so the spinal cord sends endless signals to the muscles to contract. There are many temporary ways to reduce spasticity, including medications, but there is only one way to end spasticity: re-establishing brain control over the spastic muscles.

Speed-intensive gait training (SIGT)

Gait (walking) training that is done at speeds that are faster than typical gait training. Some researchers believe walking speed and quality will improve when gait training occurs at faster speeds.

Spontaneous recovery

Recovery with little effort. **Spontaneous recovery** is usually a result of neurons "stunned" during the acute phase coming back on line during the **subacute phase**.

Stages of recovery

See Brunnström's stages of recovery.

Stretch reflex

The immediate muscle-protection reaction caused by impulses from the spinal cord. Stretch reflexes protect muscles from being over-stretched and torn. The patellar stretch reflex, in which a clinician will use a reflex hammer to tap just below the kneecap, is an example of a stretch reflex.

Stroke survivor

A person who has a stroke but does not die from the stroke.

Subluxation of the shoulder

Dislocation of the shoulder joint as the head of the humerus (upper arm bone) separates from the glenoid fossa of the scapula (shoulder blade bone). Width of separation is usually measured in fingerbreadths. Shoulder subluxation may or may not be painful.

Subacute phase

The subacute phase broadly runs from seven days to three months. It is a time of relatively rapid recovery. This rapid recovery corresponds to the resolution of the **penumbra**. For some survivors, the subacute phase can last beyond the first year.

Synergistic movement

Movement that does not allow isolated movement of just one joint, but requires the movement of all the joints in the limb in order to perform that one movement. *See also* **mass synergies** and **synergy**.

Synergy

The combination of more than one action that always happens together, usually in a complementary way. In stroke survivors, synergy, **synergistic movement**, and **mass synergies** are used to describe movements that are necessarily bundled together in a way that makes isolated movement impossible.

Task-oriented therapy

See task-specific training.

Task-specific training

The practicing of tasks that are meaningful to the stroke survivor. For instance, if a stroke survivor is a golfer, practice that involves some aspect of golf, or tasks that have the potential to lead to some aspect of the game of golf, are said to be task specific. In research with both humans and animals it has been shown that recovery efforts that incorporate tasks that are meaningful may drive neuroplastic change along with increased active movement.

Taub, Edward, PhD

The originator of **constraint-induced therapy**. Dr. Taub worked for decades with lab animals, proving that constraint-induced therapy could work prior to introducing the therapy to human populations.

Thrombolytic stroke

A stroke caused by a clot formed inside a blood vessel in the brain or leading to the brain.

Transient ischemic attack (TIA)

Just like a full-blown stroke, a TIA is interruption of blood flow to the brain. However, the blood flow stops for less than 24 hours. In most cases, blood flow is stopped for one to two hours. Symptoms resolve within 24 hours. Approximately one third of people who have had a TIA eventually have a stroke. Five percent of people will have a stroke within two days after TIA. Five percent to 10 percent of patients that have had a TIA will have a stroke within the following week. A TIA is seen as a warning sign for future stroke. It also presents an opportunity to implement lifestyle changes to reduce the chances of having a stroke.

Treadmill training (TT)

A form of gait (walking) training that incorporates a treadmill. Treadmills offer "endless parallel bars," a predictable and nonslip walking surface, and gradation of incline or speed—all with indoor safety and comfort.

Tremor

Involuntary, usually rhythmic, movements.

Unilateral spatial neglect (USN)

Also known as hemineglect, hemispatial neglect, hemiagnosia, unilateral neglect, spatial neglect, unilateral visual inattention, hemi-inattention. A survivor who has unilateral neglect is less aware or completely unaware of the affected side. Even after they are reminded to look at the hand, they often will only glance at it as if it holds little interest to them. USN can be dangerous; the survivor will bump into or ignore objects on the affected side. Sometimes USN can extend beyond the body of the survivor so that the whole space on the "bad" side of the body is ignored. Constraint-induced therapy and mirror therapy may be helpful in reducing USN.

Waist-to-hip ratio

The relationship between the measurement of the stomach and the hips. To calculate, divide the measurement around the belly by the measurement around the hips. The belly is measured at the belly button, and the hips are measured around their widest point. The calculation is:

(Waist measurement) ÷ (Hip measurement) = (Waist-to-hip ratio) There are many waist-to-hip ratio calculators on the web (Google: "waist-to-hip ratio calculator"). Research has shown that the waist-to hip ratio is one of the best indicators of cardiac (heart attack) risk.

Wolf's law

A widely accepted theory that the more stress put on a bone over time will reshape that bone to better handle that stress. Bone will get thicker and stronger if one does resistance exercises (weight training or working muscles against any resistance such as gravity or resistance bands). Stroke survivors tend to have weaker bones (osteoporosis) on the affected side, coupled with the fact that when stroke survivors fall, they tend to fall toward the affected side. Since the bones on that side are weak, there is increased risk of fracture. Wolf's law can be used to make bones thicker and stronger, reducing the risk of fracture.

Index

About the Author

Peter G. Levine is the director of SynapsTogether, dedicated to finding and reporting on the best systems for driving cortical plasticity. Since the 1990s, Pete has been involved in stroke-specific clinical research as a Research Associate first in the Human Performance & Motion Analysis Laboratory at the Kessler Institute for Rehabilitation, and more recently as a Research Associate and Co-Director of the Neuromotor Recovery and Rehabilitation Laboratory (NMRRL), Department of Rehabilitation Sciences at the University of Cincinnati. Peter continues with the NMRRL (located in the Ohio State University Medical Center) as a consultant. He has written dozens of articles for magazines and has co-authored more than 60 peer-reviewed journal articles and abstracts. Peter is also an educator, giving more than 80 stroke-specific continuing education and professional talks per year.

Pete resides in Wyoming, Ohio, with his wife, Aila Mella (a physical therapist), and their two children, Emma Maria and Jesse Martin.

Pete can be reached via e-mail at: **StrongerAfterStroke@yahoo.com**

Websites: RecoverFromStroke.blogspot.com

SynapsTogether.blogspot.com